Holy Herbs

*Modern Connections
to Ancient Plants*

Sudhir Ahluwalia

L!FE

Reprint 2023

FiNGERPRINT! L!FE
An imprint of Prakash Books India Pvt. Ltd.

113/A, Darya Ganj, New Delhi-110 002,
Tel: (011) 2324 7062 – 65, Fax: (011) 2324 6975
E-mail: info@prakashbooks.com/sales@prakashbooks.com

facebook www.facebook.com/fingerprintpublishing
twitter www.twitter.com/FingerprintP, www.fingerprintpublishing.com

ISBN: 978 81 7599 446 1

Processed & printed in India

Dedication

This is for Vibha, my wife,
without whose support
this would not have been possible.

CONTENTS

INTRODUCTION

Today, there is an increasing trend towards organic and green living worldwide. Herbal products, derived from plants and trees are extensively found in foods, nutritional supplements, cosmetics, traditional medicines, and folk remedies.

The global herbal product industry, as per Eurostat figures, reached nearly $200 billion in sales in 2005. According to Kennedy (2005), approximately 38.2 million adults aged 45–64 in the United States used herbs and supplements in 2002. The rates were higher for women than for men (21.0 percent vs. 16.7 percent, respectively).

The Chicago-based research firm, Mintel, estimated that U.S. retail sales of homeopathic and herbal remedies reached $6.4 billion in 2012, up by almost 3 percent from 2011, and has grown 16 percent over the past five years. Mintel forecasted an increase in sales, to $7.5 billion by 2017.

Many products that are popular today have a long history. Ancient texts mention the use of herbs, plants, and trees in food, cosmetics, religious rituals, and medicine. This book investigates the scientific evidence that supports or refutes traditional uses of herbal products, particularly those described in the Old and New Testaments, the *Talmud*, the *Quran*, and the *Hadiths*, which continue to influence billions of people.

By investigating these texts from a historical and scientific viewpoint, I have sought to draw connections between the past and present, as well as between the various cultures and geographies discussed herein.

The Bible, for example, is one of the greatest sources of ancient human history. It describes views, thoughts, practices, and value systems of Jews and Christians from the ancient empires of Babylon, Mesopotamia, Egypt, Persia, Macedonia, Greece, and Rome.

In particular, this book strives to answer the following questions:

1. What is the origin and correct identification of plants mentioned in important religious texts, such as the *Bible*, and secular literature?
2. What was the value of these herbs in Biblical times?
3. How was trade in herbs conducted over the millennia, and to what extent does this trade survive?
4. What archaeological evidence supports the use of herbal products?
5. What, if any, current research supports the use of herbal products?
6. Do herbal products have relevance in modern medicine, such as in the treatment of cancer, Alzheimer's disease, diabetes, high blood pressure, obesity, and so on?

Most books about herbs list various uses with no scientific explanations. They tend to promote the credentials of people who recommend these herbs, and reinforce the false view that herbal products have no side effects and are completely safe for human use.

For example, cinnamon is mentioned in the Book of Exodus in the Bible as a component of the holy anointing oil, and it continues to be a popular spice today. However, scientific analysis has revealed the presence of an alkaloid in cinnamon that can damage the liver when ingested in excess amounts.

There is also disagreement regarding the identity of many herbs mentioned in the Bible and other important religious texts. This book identifies the most probable contemporary species, and offers balanced information about the botanical origins, history, and current research.

Archaeological and documentary evidence of the use of herbs among Jews, Christians, Hindus, and Muslims from ancient Greece, Egypt, and Mesopotamia is discussed. Similarities across various cultures and regions of the Mediterranean, Northern Africa, Asia, and Europe are identified and analysed. An extensive bibliography of reference material is also provided.

The primary audience for this book includes people who are interested in herbal sciences, such as alternative medicine scholars, naturopaths, herbal product manufacturers and traders, herb growers, herbal product users, members of organic and green living communities, research scientists, and biotechnology industry professionals.

The book is organised as follows:

Chapter 1: **Historical Overview** provides background on the use and trade of herbs and spices in ancient Egypt, Mesopotamia, Greece, Rome, China, and India from the third millennium BC to the early twentieth century. Throughout history, herbal products such as pepper, frankincense, aloe, cinnamon, and cassia have been extensively traded. Three major ancient transcontinental trade routes (the Incense Route, Spice Route, and Silk Road) were used to trade herbs, spices, and wood through to the nineteenth century AD, and often evoked international conflict.

Chapter 2: **The Bible and the Herbs of the Holy Anointing Oil** discusses the origins and botanical nomenclature of herbs used in religious rituals, and focuses on the four herbs of the holy anointing oil (myrrh, calamus, cinnamon, and cassia). These herbs were imported from Northern Africa, the Arabian Peninsula, and India. Some, like cinnamon and cassia, continue to be popular today, whereas the use of myrrh and calamus has diminished.

Chapter 3: **Herbs in Ancient Incenses and Perfumes** summarises the properties and uses of several ancient incense plants (agarwood, frankincense, stacte, styrax, benzoin, galbanum, spikenard, saffron, crocus, onycha, costus, and henna). Many religions use herbs and spices in incenses and rituals, such as preparing bodies for burial. For example, herbs were used to prepare Jesus's body after his crucifixion.

Chapter 4: **Sacred Trees** explores the early periods of the Bible when trees were regarded as sacred. Modern scientific study has validated many traditional medicinal properties of products derived from these trees. In particular, this chapter discusses cedar, date palm, sycamore, olive, pomegranate, willow, and myrtle.

Chapter 5: **Culinary Herbs in the Bible** discusses ancient culinary herbs (hyssop, wormwood, rue, coriander, cumin, fitches, dill, mustard, and mint). The origin of hyssop, for example, is debated by both religious and secular scholars. Others, like dill, mustard, and mint, continue to be popular in cuisines across the globe.

Bibliograhy: provides a bibliography of reference material for each chapter.

CHAPTER 1

HISTORICAL OVERVIEW

Rock paintings in France, India, and other parts of the world show prehistoric human interaction with nature. These paintings from the Stone Age date from 30,000 years ago in Africa to 3300 BC (the start of the Bronze Age) in Eastern Asia. They show wood, nuts, leaves, berries, barks, and seeds as sources of nutrition, medicine, shelter, energy, entertainment, and beauty, and indicate that humans learned to use specific plants to enhance their food and health.

Pottery from 6,000 years ago found in Denmark and Germany shows residues of garlic mustard, fish, and meat (Saul et al., 2013). The dyes used in the rock paintings in Bhimbetka paintings in India are of plant origin, and depict the life and times of people across millennia.

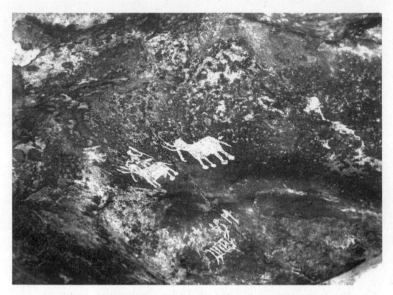

Figure 1 Bhimbetka, Madhya Pradesh, India rock paintings,
circa 30,000 BC to medieval times, own work

The *Bible, Quran, Talmud,* and other religious texts reference plants and trees extensively as sources of food, incense, flavour, medicine, and shelter. The following verse from the Bible illustrates their importance:

"The trees that are fed and nourished by the water that flows from the sanctuary have nourishing and healing properties. And by the river on its bank, on one side and on the other, will grow all [kinds of] trees for food. Their leaves will not wither, and their fruit will not fail. They will bear every month because their water flows from the sanctuary, and their fruit will be for food and their leaves for healing" (Ezekiel 47:12).

Hebrews 6:7 "For ground that drinks the rain which often falls on it and brings forth vegetation useful to those for whose sake it is also tilled, receives a blessing from God;" demonstrates the value that society placed on vegetation.

The Book of Jubilee 10:12–13 states, "As we explained to Noah all the medicines of their diseases, together with their seductions, how he might heal them with herbs of the earth. And Noah wrote down all things in a book as we instructed him concerning every kind of medicine. Thus the evil spirits were precluded from (hurting) the sons of Noah."

Sirach 38:4–5 and 7–8 states, "The Lord created medicines out of the earth and the sensible will not despise them. Was not water made sweet with a tree in order that its power might be known? . . . By them the physician heals and takes away pain; the pharmacist makes a mixture from them."

When Berodach Baladan, son of the King of Babylon, visited Hezekiah, King of Judah (c. 715–687 BC), among his most valuable possessions were spices, gold, and silver (2 Kings 20:12–14).

A handful of cardamom was worth as much as a poor man's yearly wage and slaves were bought and sold for a few cups of peppercorns. Around 1000 BC, Queen Sheba visited King Solomon in Jerusalem to offer him "120 measures of gold, many spices, and precious stones." (1 Kings 10.)

The Talmudic literature mentions approximately 70 plants used in food, spices, and medicine. Olives, dates, pomegranates, and quinces were popular fruits. Garlic, cumin, fennel flower, beet, and others were eaten as vegetables and spices. Hyssop (*Marjorana syriaca*) was used to treat intestinal worms (Shab 109 b), and beet (*Beta vulgaris*) was believed to have several medicinal properties, such as care of the eyes and bowels (Shab 133 a–f).

The Quran also makes many references to plants, herbs, and trees. Verse 61 of Surah Baqarah, for instance, states, "O Moses, we can never endure one [kind of] food. So call upon your Lord to bring forth for us from the earth its green herbs and its cucumbers and its garlic and its lentils and its onions."

THE SPICE TRADE

The five major civilisations from the fourth to the first millenniums BC were the Indus Valley Civilisation in India, the Sumerians in modern Iraq, the Egyptians, the Greeks on the isle of Crete, and the Chinese in the land north of the Himalayas.

The use of spices in food, medicine, and cosmetics began as settlements organised in the Indus Valley and across Mesopotamia from Judea, to the Nile Valley in Egypt around 9000 BC. Around the same time, livestock domestication took place in the Middle East, Hindu Kush, and western Indian plains. By 3000 BC, turmeric, cardamom, pepper, and mustard were in cultivation.

These goods and their trade were essential to the economies and cultures of these regions. The three major transcontinental trade routes included the Incense Route, the Spice Route, and the Silk Road.

The Spice Road connected India and Southeastern Asia to the Mediterranean and thus, also connected Rome, Greece, Egypt, and Africa. These regions were major producers and consumers of spices, and other luxury goods from 2500 BC to 400 BC.

The following Bible verses describe this active trade economy: "The merchants of the earth will weep and mourn over her because no one buys their cargoes anymore—12 cargoes of gold, silver, precious stones and pearls; fine linen, purple, silk and scarlet cloth; every sort of citron wood, and articles of every kind made of ivory, costly wood, bronze, iron and marble; 13 cargoes of cinnamon and spice, of incense, myrrh and frankincense, of wine and olive oil, of fine flour and wheat; cattle and sheep; horses and carriages; and human beings sold as slaves" (Revelation 18:11–13).

Prior to 400 BC, Egypt and Mesopotamia were the major powers in the region. The Incense Route, which connected the Mediterranean to the legendary Land of Punt and Arabia, was used extensively from about 700 BC to 200 AD. From the Horn of Africa and Eastern Africa came wood, feathers, animal skins, and gold. Arabia produced frankincense and myrrh.

Because of their locations on the trade routes, Middle Eastern tribes acquired prosperity. Later, as Greece's political and economic power increased, so did its appetite for luxury goods. The Romans then dominated the region from about 200 BC to 400 AD, overwhelming all major powers in the region and occupying large parts of Northern Africa and Europe.

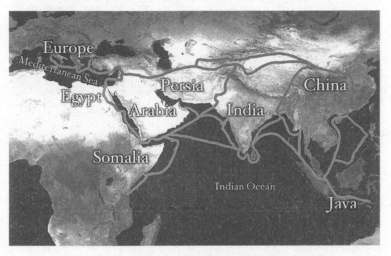

Figure 2 Spice trade routes (in blue) and Silk route (in red)

The lure of profit from the spice trade attracted European powers, who initiated exploratory expeditions. Portuguese navigator Vasco da Gama reached the western coast of India via the Cape of Good Hope in 1498. He returned with pepper and other spices, which fetched six times the cost of the expedition. This windfall led to a spurt of maritime trade between India and Europe, and intense competition among European powers for control of this trade.

Vasco da Gama's journey also led to the rediscovery of the prolific spice-producing region of the East, namely the Maluku

(Malacca) Islands. By 1511, the Portuguese controlled the spice business of the Malabar region along the western coast of India and Sri Lanka. The revenues from spices, along with West African gold, accounted for more than half of the total revenues of the Portuguese state.

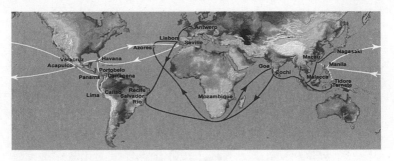

Figure 7 sixteenth century Portuguese-Spanish trade routes

The Dutch soon challenged Portuguese control over the Spice Islands (Maluku Islands), sparking a war that lasted from the fifteenth to the seventeenth centuries, and ended with the Dutch seizing control. The Dutch replaced the Portuguese and forced the local island populations to shift from agriculture to spice production. The local populace of Maluku Islands suffered hugely. Massacres were frequent.

The ecology of the Maluku Islands, a rich volcanic region, also suffered, as plantations of cloves and mace replaced native evergreen forests. The colonial powers of Europe sought to further expand the spice cultivation area into newly acquired territories in Africa and Brazil. Excess production eventually led to a supply glut and a drop in prices. The Dutch then attempted to drive up demand by reducing spice cultivation. It was in this atmosphere that the Dutch traded a small nutmeg-producing island called 'Run' in the Malacca archipelago with the English. In exchange, the English received a small territory in what is now the 'island of Manhattan' in New York.

By this time, Spain had acquired the area that now includes Chile and other neighboring lands, so it had access to silver and other minerals. Large-scale mining of silver led to a dramatic rise in the availability of bullion currency in Spain. Much of this bullion was diverted to Asia as payment for spices. Silver became the primary export from Europe, comprising nearly 75 percent of its total exports.

In addition to the long and perilous journeys that were common until the eighteenth century, limited spice production was also a primary cause for high prices. At each stage of the journey, intermediaries took a profit, thus driving up the price for the end consumer. Higher production and supply changed the supply-demand balance.

The introduction of organised corporate trading with large companies and exchanges led to a decline in the number of intermediaries. Improved storage, packaging, logistic efficiency led to lower storage costs and thus reduced risk premium. Eventually, the discovery of chemical-based alternatives for medicine and cosmetics decreased the demand for herbs. Thus, as cheaper alternatives became available, herbs and spices were no longer exclusive to the rich.

INDUS VALLEY

The Indus Valley Civilisation inhabited the flood plains and tributaries of the Indus River and the proximal coastal areas of the Arabian Sea, including most of Western India and modern day Pakistan, Iran, and Afghanistan. The Indus Valley people were famous for their planned cities, many of which have been excavated and dated, such as Mohenjo Daro and the port city of Lothal. Archeologists have excavated cities in Harappa (modern day Pakistan) that were built from 2500 to 1800 BC.

Trade between the Indus Valley and Mesopotamia, Egypt, China, and Greece has been recorded by historians, philosophers, healers, religious leaders, and politicians. Goods and services from each of these regions traveled vast distances, through forests inhabited by wild animals, deserts, and inhospitable territories.

Indus Valley seals have been recovered from settlements around the Persian Gulf. Products from India, Sri Lanka, and Indonesia included pepper, cardamom, cinnamon, nutmeg, and cloves, as well as wood, ghee (clarified butter), textiles, precious stones, and metal tools. The Epic of Gilgamesh, a collection of stories and poems discovered in Mesopotamia, and dating back to 2100 BC, mentions trade in wood, resin, cloth, and other materials. It also references the destruction of a mountain rich in cedar forests in the region that is now Lebanon. The stories are similar to the tales of the Biblical Garden of Eden and Noah's flood. This evidence points to the intimate cultural connection between Babylon and the larger Judean-Palestinian region.

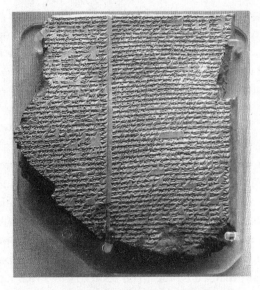

Figure 3 "British Museum Flood Tablet" by BabelStone, own work

The western coast of India, in particular, was dotted with ports from Cape Comorin to the Gulf of Cambay in Gujarat, including the oldest discovered port of Lothal (c. 2400 BC) on the Sabarmati River. Muziris, on the coast of modern Kerala, was a popular port for exporting to Mediterranean countries. Its monsoonal climate is well suited for cultivation of evergreens, cinnamon, cardamom, sandalwood, and teak. Pepper has been cultivated for thousands of years in the Malabar region.

Nutmeg and cloves came from the Maluku Islands (Malacca Islands) and Spice Islands, which are part of Indonesia and Sri Lanka today. Sri Lanka continues to be a major producer and exporter of cinnamon.

Eastern India also had several ports for trading with Arabian, Mesopotamian, Chinese, and Mediterranean regions. Goods were transported directly to China by sea, and to the Mediterranean via the straits of Malacca, then north along the coastline to the Persian Gulf. Further transport through the Middle East, and on to Europe was by land. Another route took the goods by boat via the Persian Gulf to Mesopotamia, and by land through Palestine, Egypt, and Europe. It was common for goods to take a full year to reach their destination.

Cultural Influence of Indus Valley

The Indus Valley was a transition zone from 530 BC to the third century AD. Rulers such as Cyrus the Great (538–530 BC), Darius 1 (521–486 BC), Alexander the Great (c. 325 BC), and empires such as the Mauryan, Seleucid, and Kushan Empires (second century BC to third century AD) linked the history and cultures of the surrounding regions.

To the west was Assyria, Mesopotamia, Palestine, Judea, Greece, Rome, and Europe. To the north was China and the central Asian regions. To the east was the Indian subcontinent and Maluku Islands.

There were peaceful times, such as during the Seleucid Kingdom, and there were disruptions caused by invasions and geopolitical events. The modern term "globalisation" also applies to this period of human history, when scholars, kings, traders, and religious people sought conquest, trade, culture, and religious enlightenment.

Records from the Mauryans (322–185 BC) show that spices used at that time included salts (e.g., table, rock, sea, bida, nitre) and spices (e.g., long pepper, cumin, coriander, cloves, turmeric, mustard).

Kashyap and Weber (2010) conducted studies at Farmana, an Indus Valley civilisation burial site close to Delhi in modern India, and found turmeric, ginger, and garlic cloves in food prepared around 2500 BC. McIntosh (2008) indicated that the Harappans probably consumed spices like mustard, coriander, mango, caper, garlic, turmeric, ginger, cumin, and cinnamon, all of which were locally available. Sesame, and probably linseed oil were used as cooking oils. Grinding stones, which were used to pound grain and spices, have also been discovered in excavations of the Indus Valley.

In ancient Indian tradition, the *Vedas* (c. 1500 BC) are sacred writings containing chants used in rituals and daily life to propitiate the gods. The use of herbs, plants, and spices in Ayurvedic medicine has been extensively documented. For example, the *Vedas* mention a holy fire ritual called *Yagnya*, in which people lit fires and chanted verses to appease Agni, the god of fire, and other gods. Rituals, chants, and herbs formed an integral part of medical treatment.

Sushruta and Charaka, two renowned surgeons of ancient India, compiled s*amhitas*, or compilations, of medicinal practices, from the sixth century BC onwards. These works mention imported and indigenous herbs and spices that treat a range of ailments. They also include herbal recipes for disease prevention and cosmetics.

Based on an analysis of archaeological evidence gathered from previous Indus Valley civilisation sites, many herbs and plants mentioned in Ayurveda were also used in the Indus Valley period (c. 2800–1500 BC).

MESOPOTAMIA AND THE SUMERIANS

The ancient Mesopotamia region comprises modern Iraq, Iran, Israel, Palestine, Syria, and Turkey. For more than 5,000 years, the Mesopotamia region rivaled the great powers of India, China, Egypt, Greece, and Rome. The lands of Mesopotamia formed a bridge between the eastern civilisations of India and China and the western civilisations of Greece, Rome, and Egypt.

The first historical evidence of Mesopotamia can be traced back to 3500 BC. The region was divided into the principalities of Sumer and other small kingdoms. Over its long history, the region was influenced and dominated by the Assyrians, Greeks, Parthians, Romans, and Iranians. Soon after the death of the Prophet Muhammad, the region became part of the Muslim caliphate. The Mongols then controlled Mesopotamia from 1215 to 1453 AD, and the Ottoman Empire reigned from 1450 until the 1900s.

The Mesopotamia-Persian region was strategically located along the ancient Silk Road and the Incense Route. Mesopotamia was a consumer, trader, producer, and exporter of herbs, spices, agricultural commodities, and other goods. The common spices used in the region included coriander, saffron, garlic, pepper, mint, myrrh, cedar, laurel, sage, basil, oregano, rosemary, and dill.

The *Assyrian Herbal*, first published in 1924, compiled information from 660 clay tablets of Babylonian medical texts (c. 2000–3000 BC). It describes 250 medicinal substances, including spices like fennel, myrrh, saffron, and turmeric, many of which were imported from Asia.

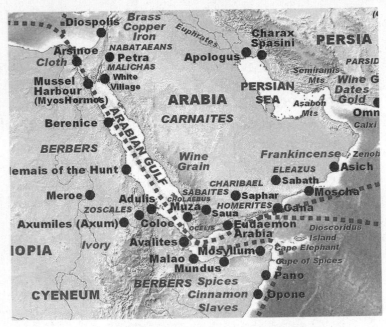

Figure 4 Arabia and the region according to Periplus
Maris Erythaei (circa first century AD)

In 1772 BC, the *Code of Hammurabi*, which was enacted during
the reign of King Hammurabi and encoded Mesopotamian
governance practices, was inscribed on stone steles and clay
tablets. The Code of Hammurabi shared common elements with
other Mesopotamia codes, like the *Code of Ur Nammu* (c. 2050
BC), *Laws of Eshnunna* (c. 1930 BC), and *Code of Lipit-Ishtar of
Ishin* (c. 1870 BC). The Code of Hammurabi is perhaps the most
comprehensive in terms of detail, and extensive in terms of its
reach in Mesopotamia.

The Code of Hammurabi contains specific medical
instructions. For example, surgeons were permitted to practice
medicine but were bound by the code of an "eye for an eye"
which meant that a surgeon could lose his limb, eye, etc. in case a

patient were to suffer damage as a consequence of the treatment. Thus, injuring a patient could lead to serious punishment.

This discouragement of surgical science may have led to the popularity of herbal medicine. Around 250 plants, 120 minerals, and another 180 other drugs are mentioned in medical literature of the time. The oldest Babylonian medical text known today is the *Esagil-kin-apli* (c. 1069–1046 BC), or *Diagnostic Handbook*, which lists medical practices and prescriptions of the Hammurabi era, including herbs, incenses, and spices that are still in use today.

Sumerians lived in modern day Iraq. Uruk was one of the largest Sumerian cities, with a population of 80,000. Cuneiform tablets that date back to 3000 BC offer some information about this civilisation. These clay tablets refer to odoriferous plants, including thyme. Some of these spices, like cardamom, were imported from Sri Lanka, India, and China. The tablets also contain extensive references to the cultivation and use of plants in Mesopotamia. For example, onions were grown in the first millennium but were probably reserved for the elite, as there was an office that regulated onion distribution.

A tablet from the Yale Babylonian collection mentions extensive use of herbs and spices in cuisine. Sesame and olive oils appear to be popular Sumerian cooking oils around 2200 BC. Herbs were also an important source of perfumes, incense, and cosmetics. Perfume makers operated in the Mesopotamian Palace of Mari, in the modern city of Tel Hariri in Syria, as early as 1800 BC. The Persians produced essential oils from roses, lilies, and coriander. Saffron, too, was in great demand.

Around 722 BC, the King of Assyria and Babylon, Merodach Baladan, owned a garden with sixty-one species of herbs and spices, such as coriander, cress, black cumin, fennel, mustard, licorice, juniper berries, mint, dill, safflower, thyme, hyssop, and asafoetida. One source states that the harvesting of the spices from this garden was done on moonlit nights only, for it was believed that this would preserve the potency of the herbs.

King Ashurbanipal of Assyria (668–633 BC) also recorded a long list of aromatic plants like thyme, sesame, cardamom, turmeric, saffron, poppy, garlic, cumin, anise, coriander, silphium, dill, and myrrh. Onions, garlic, and shallots were popular condiments in Persia in the sixth century BC. King Cyrus (559–529 BC) is said to have purchased 395,000 bundles of garlic.

Arabian tribes controlled the Red Sea ports and desert land routes of the Mediterranean region. Before the domestication of camels around 900 BC, donkeys were used on these slow and ponderous routes. Petra, in modern Jordan, was an important trading station on this route from Africa and India to Egypt, Greece, Rome, and Europe. When Alexander conquered Egypt in the fourth century BC, access to the markets of Europe shifted to the port of Alexandria. Eventually, Alexandria became the most important of the Red Sea ports and a major center for the trade of spices, incense, and other goods.

Cultural Influence of Mesopotamia and Islam

A dynamic and new religion, Islam, came into being in the seventh century in the Arabian Peninsula. Arabia was a major trade hub, linking India, China, and Africa with the Mediterranean powers of Greece, Egypt, and Rome, and eventually the emerging markets of Europe. Thus, Arabia rapidly expanded its influence across Asia, Europe, and Africa. Arab scholars translated the medical works of Greek scholars.

The Persian preference for rice, nuts, honey, and sweets was adopted throughout the Arabian Peninsula, Southern Europe, and Southern and Central Asia. During this age of dynamism, many scholars of Arab medicine emerged, such as Al Tabbari (838–870), Al Razi (Rhazes) (846–930), Al Zahrawi (930–1013),

Ibn Sina or Avicenna (980–1037), Ibn Al Haitham (960–1040), Ibn Al Nafees (1213–1288), and Ibn Khaldun (1332–1395).

Ibn Sina authored a magnum opus, the *Canon of Medicine*, which was translated into Latin in the twelfth century, and dominated the medical world for centuries. The second volume of the *Canon of Medicine* lists 235 remedies, including 760 medicinal plants and their uses.

The search for new cures from the herbal world was further fueled by the teaching of Prophet Muhammad, who said, "God has provided a remedy for every illness." (Bashar Saad, Omar Said 2011) Muslim scholars added herbs from the Arabian Peninsula, India, Persia, and China to the list of remedies.

New drugs introduced by Arabs included senna, camphor, sandalwood, cassia, tamarind, nutmeg, and aconite, in addition to the existing ones like myrrh and cloves. New ways of administering medicine were developed, including elixirs, pills, tinctures, suppositories, inhalations, syrups, juleps, and more palatable solvents such as rosewater and orange blossom water, which could replace unguents and healing oils. The Arab pharmacopoeia included herbs and spices from vast territories of China, Persia, India, Southeastern Asia, and Northern and Eastern Africa.

Arabic physicians emphasised the importance of trials, experiments, and observation-based medicine. Abu Bakr Rhazes (846–930 AD) used animals to test the safety and efficacy of medicines. The first test subject, a monkey, was used to test the effects of mercury on the human body. These studies can be described as the earliest of clinical trials.

Arab influence continued until the nineteenth century, when synthetic drugs replaced herbal medicines and the center of drug discovery and medicine shifted to Europe. However, even today, as organic and natural alternatives become more popular, Arabic medicine continues to be an affordable alternative for millions worldwide.

The Arab Union for Agriculture and Development (2000) reports that, out of 814 plant species used in traditional Arab medicine, twenty-three are still in use in the pharmaceutical industry, fifty-five in the skin care and perfume industries, thirty-four in the food industry, and ten in the botanical pesticide industry.

EGYPT

The earliest dynasties of Egypt date back to the second half of the fourth millennium BC. Ancient Egyptians used spices and herbs to provide nutritional benefit. Queen Hatshepsut of Egypt (c. 1458 BC) sent a flotilla of six Egyptian ships to the Land of Punt (on the eastern coast of Africa) to buy such goods. Hieroglyphs show ships laden with goods and cedar tree plants docked in the port of Egypt. Cedar plants from Eastern Africa were highly valued, and the Queen commissioned ships to bring them to Egypt, and plant them locally.

Archaeologists and anthropologists have discovered evidence of the use of coriander, garlic, cassia, myrrh, frankincense, and salt in ancient Egypt from 3500 BC onwards. Hieroglyphs show pyramid workers eating onions and garlic, which was thought to give them additional strength and to prevent digestive ailments. Pharaonic Egyptians were known to use anise, marjoram, fenugreek, mustard, cumin, fennel, salt, dill, sesame, nutmeg, and coriander.

The concept of an afterlife after death was an important belief of ancient Egyptians. Preserving the dead through mummification was common among the rich and mighty. Mummification involved desiccating the body with salt after disemboweling it. The cavity was then filled with sweet smelling myrrh.

The Greek historians Herodotus (484 BC-425BC) described the mummification processes in Egypt. Jars filled with spices, herbs, and valuables were buried in the tomb with the dead, because it was thought that the dead person should have the best things available for use in the afterlife. Herbs, trees, and spices were among the most valuable of commodities of that time. A mural on the temple walls of Egyptian Queen Hatshepsut (1458 BC) depicts sacks of frankincense.

Cultural Influence of Egypt

Ancient Egypt was the most advanced society of its time with the most renowned physicians. Anyone with the means in the second millennium BC or later, could come to Egypt for treatment. This type of travel is not very different from the medical tourism that exists today.

There was intense interaction between the ancient Egyptians and Greeks. Scholars from Greece would often visit Egypt to learn about their medicinal practices. Greek historian Herodotus wrote of Egypt: "The practice of medicine is very specialised among them. Each physician treats just one disease. The country is full of physicians, some treat the eye, some the teeth, some of what belongs to the abdomen and others internal diseases" (Histories 2, 84). Imhotep, who is regarded as the earliest Egyptian herbal physician, was revered by the Egyptians and Greeks as a god of medicine. Trade between the ancient Indians and Egyptians dates back to at least the third century BC.

Egyptian texts contain many references to herbs, including frankincense, myrrh, cedar, balsam, pine, myrtle, benzoin, labdanum, mastic, juniper berry, cardamom, and calamus. Many of these herbs were ingredients in Kyphi (known as *Kapet* in ancient Egypt), an antiseptic, perfumed substance that was used extensively in ancient Egyptian temples and the homes of the rich. *Papyrus Harris*, written during the reign of Rameses IV (c. 1155–1149 BC), contains a recipe for Kyphi. According to the Ebers papyrus, Kyphi was sprinkled liberally in tombs of pharaohs to be enjoyed in the afterlife.

Many Egyptian papyri have survived, and they are valuable resources about Egyptian medicine and the importance of herbs (www.reshafim.org.il/ad/egypt). These include the Edwin Smith papyrus; Kahun Gynaecological papyrus; Berlin Medical papyrus; London Medical papyrus; Hearst Medical papyrus (which contains many of the same recipes as those in the Ebers papyrus); and the Demotic Magical Papyrus of London and Leiden.

The oldest papyrus, the Ebers papyrus, dates back to 1550 BC. The Ebers papyrus discusses medicinal herbs used by ancient Egyptian doctors dating back to 3400 BC. Ebers was a German Egyptologist and novelist who purchased the ancient papyrus record in 1873. The papyrus, which resides at the University of Leipzig in Germany, lists 876 herbs and 500 plants.

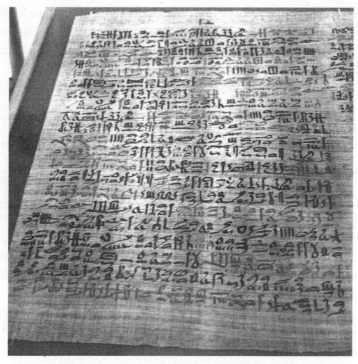

Figure 5 The Ebers papyrus (c. 1550 BC) from ancient Egypt,
Einsamer Schützederivative work

Exorcisms, spells, and herbal remedies were the main tools for healing. Incantations, prayers (particularly to Sekhmet, the goddess of healing) played important roles. The wearing of amulets and the importance of diet were emphasised: herbs alleviated pain only, whereas magic cured.

The Ebers papyrus states, "Magic is effective together with medicine. Medicine is effective together with magic." It mentions opium, cannabis, myrrh, frankincense, fennel, cassia, senna, thyme, henna, juniper, aloe, and linseed, and castor oil. Many, like castor and juniper, were locally available; others were imported from Africa and Asia (e.g., mandrake, cedar oil, henna, aloe, and frankincense).

The Greeks and Romans translated the Egyptian texts into their languages. Over the centuries, Greek and Roman texts became the basis of Arabic and European medical texts.

GREECE AND ROME

By 2500 BC, a civilisation had emerged on the island of Crete in the Aegean Sea. The region was likely settled by Minoans even earlier, around 3000 BC. Around the sixteenth or seventeenth century BC, a volcanic eruption of the Santorini volcano led to the sudden destruction of the Minoan society. The great Minoan cities lay covered under a cloud of volcanic dust until they were uncovered in the twentieth century by Sir Arthur Evans (1851-1941), a British archaeologist. His excavations have revealed grand palaces and ship wrecks that indicate an active sea trade in the Mediterranean region, most likely with Egypt, Canaan (modern Lebanon and Syria), Arabia, and Judea.

In 325 BC, the Greek empire expanded from the Persian region to the Indus Valley, increasing use of the Silk Route connecting China and central Asia to Greece, and beyond. Many Greek philosophers of the time recorded their thoughts and observations.

Megasthenes (c. 350–290 BC), the Greek Ambassador to the court of the Mauryan Emperor Chandragupta, observed that exports and imports consisted mostly of incense, spices, textiles, silk, metals, glassware, and slaves. Megasthenes and Pliny the Elder (23–79 AD), the Roman author and naturalist, mentioned Muziris (now the Indian state of Kerala), the spice-producing region and most popular port on the western coast of India.

Pliny the Elder also mentions the southern Indian kingdom and trade center of Pandya (modern day Tamil Nadu in Southern India), which was ruled by a succession of kings from about 600 BC to 1700 AD. Pandyan ports were transit ports for the spice trade between Southeastern Asia and Red Sea Egyptian ports that were then controlled by Imperial Rome. Strabo (64 BC–23 AD) mentions that the Pandyan King had diplomatic relations with Augustus Caesar.

Hippalus was a Greek sailor in the first century AD who may have been the first mariner to discover a direct route from India to the Red Sea. Ships used the annual monsoon winds to undertake a rapid transit across the Indian Ocean. This shorter and speedier route benefited the global trade business. When the monsoon currents reversed, sailors journeyed back from Arabia to India. The first leg took about ten days, whereas the trip back took nearly a year to complete. Other scholars claim that the monsoon trade route was discovered by Arabs much earlier, around the first century AD.

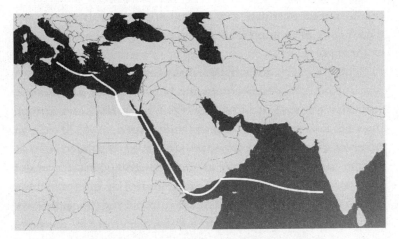

Figure 6 "Italy to India Route" by Morn, own work

Romans were major consumers of spices. As the center of consumption moved westwards with the rise of the Roman Empire, Mediterranean ports (e.g., Carthage in modern Tunisia) became prominent. Gold and silver coins were used as currency, as indicated by discovery of Roman gold and silver coins from the first century AD in excavations by the Archaeological Survey of India, and villagers off and on, both on the western and eastern coasts of Southern India.

As the cost of spices in Roman ports increased to a hundred times more than their market value, and as the supply of spices from India increased, a trade imbalance occurred between Greece, Rome, and India. Pliny the Elder estimated this imbalance to be 20 million denarii (perhaps as much as US $3.2 million), a huge sum for those times. Most trade occurred from the Southwestern Indian ports located along the Indian Ocean. India exported spices, herbs, clarified butter, timber, and textiles into Roman lands. Rome exported gold, silver, and glassware to India.

This active trade continued until about the sixth century AD, when the Roman Empire declined, and the European trade center moved westward to Constantinople (now Istanbul), and then Venice. The entire European region was eventually served by these ports.

The rise of Islamic empires in the Middle East and Western Asia further challenged commerce between India and Europe until Mongol invasions in Persia, the Middle East, and Europe stopped it altogether. Ottoman rule began in 1300 AD in Anatolia (modern Turkey) and gradually expanded to the Middle East, Europe, and Egypt. Constantinople came under Ottoman control in 1453, and thus control of the spice trade shifted to the Ottomans. Political turmoil and transport risk led to a reduction in trade, and a sharp increase in the price of spices. A pound of nutmeg in Europe thus became more valuable than gold.

Cultural Influence of Greece and Rome

The dominance of the Greeks and then Romans influenced life, culture, food, and practices of the entire region from North Africa to West Europe. Spices were used extensively in regional cuisines. Those who could afford the expensive imported herbal products like pepper, cinnamon, nutmeg, and others used them in food, cosmetics, and medicine. Others used local herbs like dill, coriander, and rosemary in food and drink.

Early Greeks regarded Mother Nature as a healing goddess. Aesculapius, the son of Apollo, was the Greek god of healing. Greeks regarded illness as a form of divine punishment, and healing as a gift from God. The basis of Greek medicine was the body's natural ability to heal itself (*pepsis*). Modern nutritional and lifestyle therapy, with its emphasis on diet and exercise, evolved in part from ancient Greek and Roman traditions. It was also a prevailing belief that social status and gender were important in healing. The rich had better access to healthy food and leisure, and were thus healthier.

Greco-Roman medicine is called Unani. The earliest Greek medical school, Knidos School, was founded around 700 BC at Knidos. Hippocrates (c. 470–360 BC), regarded as the Father of Medicine, later opened his medical school at Kos. Hippocrates travelled widely, collecting plants, learning from local practices, and using plants for various healing purposes. These were recorded in a systematic manner.

He used observation and reason as opposed to religion for answers. He insisted that priests and healers live separately. He also looked to the patient's environment for cures. Hippocrates thus created a holistic medicine based on the human body, and he emphasised the use of available therapies.

The idea that diseases have natural, and not divine causes, was a critical evolution in Hippocratic medicine. The emergence of regimens for diet, exercise, humors (body fluids), and purging can all be attributed to Hippocratic medicine. Purging included bloodletting, emetics, laxatives, diuretics, and enemas.

Hippocrates said, "Let your food be medicine and your medicine be food." He believed in a balance between environment and lifestyle, and many of these concepts remain relevant today.

Herbal medicine began around the time that one of Aristotle's students, Theophrastus (c. 371–287 BC), began observing nature, especially the habits and attributes of plants and animals. Theophrastus classified 540 animal species and wrote a series of books on botany, nine of which survive. They describe plants like pepper, cinnamon, myrrh, frankincense, banyan, and a number of local Greek plants. He relied on his own observations, as well as those of travelers, such as visitors from Asia during the reign of Alexander the Great. His work *Historia Plantarum* is regarded as one of the most important contributions of antiquity to botany.

As Greek doctors moved or were summoned to the service of Rome, the center of modern medicine shifted there. Galen (c. 129 AD) was a Greek surgeon and Roman citizen who served as a doctor in the Roman army. He enjoyed botany and collected plants during his travels. Pliny's work *Historia Naturalis* describes medical uses for more than one thousand plants.

It is regarded as a seminal work in medicine and one of the first texts to standardise drug manufacturing.

In the late eleventh century, a series of translations of the Classical texts, mainly from Arabic but also from the original Greek, revived the Hippocratic-Galenic tradition in the West. During the Renaissance, more translations of Galen and Hippocrates, directly from the Greek (Byzantine manuscripts), became available.

Dioscorides (c. 40–90 AD) was a Roman army surgeon whose writing on herbal medicine served as a textbook for 1,500 years. His book, *De Materia Medica*, describes 600 herbs and formed the basis of Western pharmacopoeia until the nineteenth century. The influence of this work on European herbal medicine eclipsed that of the *Hippocratic Corpus*. He mentions the use of aromatic oils and ointments from plants like cardamom, cassia, senna, garlic, leek, cinnamon, balm of Gilead, hops, mastic, onion, caper, mustard, liquorice, caraway, cumin, parsley, lovage, and fennel.

Romans were particularly concerned with hygiene and preferred clean and antiseptic environments. Many spa complexes with hostels, baths, and gymnasia were built around thermal and naturalised springs. They built baths and flushing toilets in towns and military forts. They also built aqueducts to provide clean water to Rome, some of which are still in use today.

Plants were attributed many mythical properties and regarded as important symbols. Romans added them to wines, balms, oils, bath treatments, poultices, and healing plasters. They hung anise near their pillows to prevent bad dreams, aid digestion, and prevent epileptic attacks. They regarded basil as a symbol of love and fertility. Bay leaves were said to bring good luck and ward off evil.

European judges burnt rosemary in the courtroom to protect themselves from illnesses brought by prisoners. Decorative laurel wreaths were used to crown victors of battles, jousts, and games. Saffron-filled pillows were used to treat hangovers. Aromatic spices were strewn along funeral paths. The rich used eastern fragrances as perfumes and as scents in their oil lamps. Cinnamon imported from Sri Lanka and India was valued for its aroma and regarded as sacred.

Apicius, a food connoisseur in the fourth or fifth century AD, wrote ten recipe books that used imported Indian spices like pepper, turmeric, and ginger, as well as local spices like anise, basil, caraway, coriander, fennel, garlic, bay leaves, cumin, dill, parsley, marjoram, and poppy seed. Pepper was particularly prized and even used as currency to pay rents and taxes in Europe. When Attila the Hun attacked Rome in the fourth century AD, it is said he demanded a tribute of 3,000 pounds of pepper as payment for not sacking the city.

CHINA

In the North of the Indus Valley, and across the Himalayas, lay the kingdoms of China, with their unique focus on learning, innovation, science, and politics. An active trade between the Chinese Han empires and the people of Malacca accounted for most imported spices, such as cloves, nutmeg, and mace, which came from the Indonesian producers of the Maluku Islands. Additional trade routes through the Malacca straits to the eastern ports of India, south to Sri Lanka, and north to Cape Comorin in Western India and the Middle East allowed trade with Greece, Egypt, and Rome. This trade was largely conducted by the Malay, Chinese, Indians, Arabs, and Africans. However, China itself was not a major exporter of spices.

Cultural Influence of China

The Chinese have used herbs for thousands of years in many applications. The Chinese herbal healing system dates back to ancient times and continues to be a vibrant industry today. More than 300 herbs are listed in Chinese herbalogy. The earliest known references to plants as medicine in China appear in Shen Nung's treatise, *Classic Herbal* (c. 2625 BC). In his *Analects*, Confucius (551–479 BC) mentions ginger as a food ingredient.

Chinese courtiers around 300 BC carried cloves in their mouths as a breath freshener in the presence of the emperor. The Chinese province Kweilin was named after the *kwei* (cassia) forests that grew extensively in 216 BC. Cassia was cheaper than cinnamon, and it serves as a cinnamon substitute even today. In the fifth century AD, Chinese ships carried ginger plants to preserve food and prevent scurvy.

Another famous Chinese medicine text, *Huangdi Neijing* (*The Yellow Emperor's Classic of Internal Medicine*), dates to the Han Dynasty (c. 206 BC–220 AD). It recommends food based on health and environmental conditions. The central principal of this work is to maintain balance of qi (life force), yin, and yang. For example, in cold weather, when qi is low and yin is high, yang foods are recommended. In summer, when yin levels are low and yang is high, yin foods should be eaten.

Traditional Chinese medicine divides herbs into four categories: cool, cold, warm, and hot. Hot and warm herbs treat illnesses that are classified as cool or cold, and vice versa. Food flavours are divided into sweet, sour, pungent, and bitter. Bitter herbs have cooling properties, and thus can treat cases of accumulated body heat resulting from inadequate rest. Pungent tasting herbs have a dispersing effect on the body and thus treat 'flu conditions.

AMERICAS

Native American and South American folk culture precedes the European colonization of these regions. Like other ancient societies, they drew sustenance and inspiration from herbs, plants, trees, and nature. North American tribes followed a comprehensive healing principle in which body, mind, and spirit were treated holistically, an approach that has commonalities with the healing principles of Ayurveda, Unani, and Traditional Chinese medicines.

American Indians shared some common traits with other regions of the world. For example, they used the same plants, such as *Mentha piperita*, wormwood, aloe vera, ginseng, *Glycyrrhiza glabra* (licorice), cedar, and pine. *Acorus calamus*, mentioned in the Bible as calamus, was an important medicinal plant of North America. They also used dance and ritual in healing. Strands of this thinking can be seen in the works of the earliest Greek scholars, like Hippocrates.

In India, the Vedas too emphasised using chants to heal. Similar traditions existed in Egypt, where magic and chants were integral to healing. There were also differences. Ancient Eurasian civilisations used grains, fruits, vegetables, and spices extensively and small quantities of sea food and meat. North American Indian food was heavy in meat, with little or no spices. Local fruits like blueberries, cranberries, strawberries, wild persimmon, wild plums, acorns, nuts, and corn were extensively eaten. Moreover, whereas ancient Asian and Middle Eastern civilisations interacted with other cultures through conquest and trade, vast oceans divided the Americas from the Eurasian continents.

About 400 tribes lived in the forests and vast lands of Latin America, including the urban empires of the Incas and the Mayas. People in these regions depended on the rich bounty of the tropical soils and temperate mountain regions. Corn, cassava, tomatoes, chilies, pineapple, papaya, guava, mango, coconut, passion fruit, cheese, fish, and guinea pigs provided nutrition for the local people.

The rain forests yielded herbs, trees, and plants to use in drinks and medicine. Cocoa beans (*Theobroma cacao*) and guayusa (*Ilex guayusa*) leaves were an important source of antioxidants and caffeine. Other forest fruit, like Camu camu (*Myrciaria dubia*), were rich sources of vitamin C. Bark of cat's claw (*Uncaria tomentosa*), cat's claw (*Iridullia catigua*), and many others were used in medicine. These tribal traditions have since eroded as a result of conquest and immigration that displaced the indigenous populations of the Americas. European immigrants brought new knowledge and traditions, but protecting the heritage of these lands continues to be a challenge.

CHAPTER 2

THE BIBLE AND THE HERBS OF THE HOLY ANOINTING OIL

～∽◇∽～

As one of the most researched of ancient literatures, the Bible is a window into the life and practices of the people who lived in Israel and bordering nations of Egypt, Mesopotamia, Greece, Rome, and Judea. The Bible and other texts from that time offer a broad view of life from around 1300 BC onwards, including accounts of global trade, commerce, science, food, medicine, and culture.

The Jewish people, who were the original writers of the Bible, had lived in all the major ancient civilisations, except China, from 3000 BC. Archaeological and documented history suggests that Jews lived in harmony with the Egyptians during the time of the pharaohs and subsequent conquerors of Mesopotamia, Rome, and Persia. Simon Schama's book, *Story of the Jews* (2013) is one of the latest pieces of literature that describes the life of Jews during the pharaonic times.

The original text of the Bible was perhaps written in Hebrew and Aramaic, and later, translated into Greek. The first verses in the Old Testament may have been written around 1875 BC, when it is said that Abraham was called to Canaan (modern Lebanon). During the centuries before and after Christ, from the second century BC to the eighth century AD, the Mediterranean region was the chief center of political and economic power in the Western world.

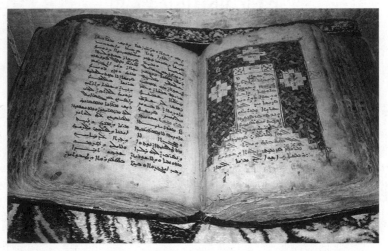

Figure 8 Bible written in Aramaic, photo courtesy of Sylvia Beth Yakub

Like other religious scriptures, the Bible emphasises the importance of plants: "And God said, Behold, I have given you every herb bearing seed, which *is* upon the face of all the earth, and every tree, in which *is* the fruit of a tree yielding seed; to you it shall be for meat" (Genesis 1:29).

Herbs and spices had immense value and were given as gifts to kings, and as tribute to temples. Queen Sheba and others brought gifts of spices and precious commodities to King Solomon and other rulers: "And she gave the king 120 talents of gold, large quantities of spices, and precious stones. Never again were so many spices brought in as those the queen of Sheba gave to King Solomon" (1 Kings 10:10).

The use of herbs and spices to flavour food is also mentioned in the Bible: "So heap on the wood and kindle the fire. Cook the meat well, mixing in the spices and let the bones be charred" (Ezekiel 24:10).

Herbs and spices had religious significance. The Bible describes rubbing Jesus' body with herbs and spices: "Taking Jesus' body, the two of them wrapped it, with the spices, in strips of linen. This was in accordance with Jewish burial customs" (John 19:40).

Herbs were used in incense, cosmetics, and perfume. The concentrated Jewish incense, *Ketoret*, is described in the Talmud, and used to prepare the Jewish temple for worship. Ketoret contains 11 ingredients: balsam (or stacte), onycha, galbanum, frankincense, myrrh, cassia, spikenard, saffron, costus, aromatic bark (perhaps cedar), and cinnamon.

Inevitably, these valuable commodities became associated with wealth, such as that of Hezekiah, the 13th King of Judah (c. 715–686 BC): "Hezekiah had very great wealth and honor, and he made treasuries for his silver and gold and for his precious stones, spices, shields and all kinds of valuables" (2 Chronicles 32:27).

In Judaism, the tabernacles (i.e., the Jewish *sanctum sanctorum*) were anointed with scented oils. This practice dates back to at least the time of Moses' exodus from Egypt (c. 1875 BC). Anointment of the head with oil was forbidden to all except clergy, though the practice was eventually extended to kings and emperors.

Many of the plants and herbs used in these ceremonies were imported at great cost from India and Africa, while others were locally produced. The Holy Anointing Oil contained pure olive oil and four spices: myrrh, cinnamon, cassia, and calamus. The specific composition is as follows: myrrh, 500 shekels (about 1 gallon); cinnamon, 250 shekels; calamus, 250 shekels; cassia, 500 shekels; olive oil, 1 hin (about $1^1/_3$ gallons). Exodus, and other verses of the Old Testament, have used the words "sweet" and "pure" when referring to these spices. Scholars have interpreted sweet to mean fragrant, and pure to mean high clarity and quality.

Christians adopted the practice of anointing the liturgy with holy anointment oil, as described in the following verse about the anointment of the Messiah: "Even though I walk through the valley of the shadow of death, I fear no evil, for You are with me; Your rod and Your staff, they comfort me. You prepare a table before me in the presence of my enemies; You have anointed my head with oil; My cup overflows. Surely goodness and loving kindness will follow me all the days of my life, And I will dwell in the house of the LORD forever" (Psalm 23:4–6).

Unlike in Judaism, anointing with oil is not an obligatory practice for Christians. The New Testament makes only four references to the use of oil. In Mark 6:13, the disciples anoint the sick, and heal them. In James 5:14, church elders anoint the sick with oil for healing.

This chapter focuses on the four herbs in the Holy Anointing Oil: myrrh, calamus, cinnamon, and cassia. These plants contain gums or resins, which help protect the plant body. Harvesting of gums and resins can be done in several ways, all of which result in wounding of the skin and revealing the gum containing channels below the bark. The gums and resins exude from the stems, branches, and rhizome (underground stem) when the plant is injured, naturally or artificially. As they harden, they seal the wound and prevent entry of pathogenic bacteria and fungi.

These gums and resins are also collected for use in herbal preparations. However, repeated depletion of gums and resins by tapping of the plant for commercial and other purpose leads to loss of plant vigor and reduction in life span of the plant.

MYRRH

Myrrh is the aromatic gum or resin that exudes from the stems and branches of more than 150 species in the Commiphora genus of the Burseraceae family (e.g., *Commiphora myrrha, Commiphora molmol, Commiphora gileadensis*). These species, which are rare today, are distributed across Eastern Africa and the Arabian Peninsula, including Ethiopia, Eritrea, Yemen, and Somalia.

C. myrrha, which is regarded as the most popular source of myrrh, grew abundantly in this region. Like other desert species around the world, the plants are leafless for much of the year. The yellowish red resin oozes from the stem, either naturally, or from artificially induced wounds. It has a bitter taste and a sweet smell.

Africa has around 50 species of Commiphora (e.g., *Commiphora abyssinica, Commiphora foliacea, Commiphora playfairii*) that yield an oleoresin, which is often mixed with the other species mentioned previously. Other species, such as *Commiphora wightii* and *Commiphora africana*, were sources of low-quality oleoresin products called bdellium and Indian myrrh. Both myrrh and bdellium belong to the same class of resins.

Myrrh was a highly prized and valuable plant. In India, the *Sushruta Samhita* mentions the use of myrrh as a herbal medicine. Chandranandan translated Sushruta Samhita into Tibetan in the eighth century AD. According to Pliny, myrrh was the royal perfume of the Parthian Empire, which encompassed modern day Iran, Iraq, and neighbouring territories. Ancient Egyptian papyrus writings from 2000 BC mention using myrrh to embalm the dead. Burning myrrh was a popular method to prevent fleas and odors.

In ancient Rome, the price for myrrh was five times that of frankincense. Herodotus references the use of myrrh as a disinfectant, an incense, and a medicine in Greece during the fifth century BC. Myrrh was burnt in funeral pyres to mask the smell.

Nero apparently burnt vast quantities of myrrh and cinnamon, a year's supply by some accounts, for his wife Poppaea's funeral.

In Traditional Chinese Medicine, myrrh was imported from the Persian region via the Silk Road, and thought to be useful to improve circulation and to treat arthritis, rheumatism, and uterine disorders.

The Talmud (Keritot 6a) describes the following incense recipe: seventy manehs of balm, onycha, galbanum, and frankincense; sixteen manehs of myrrh, cassia, spikenard, and saffron; twelve costus; three aromatic rinds; nine manehs of cinnamon nine; and lye obtained from nine leek kabs. It further specifies that if Cyprus wine is not available, old white wine may be used instead. Salt of Sodom, and an herb to make the incense smoke rise were then added in minute quantities.

The Bible contains three prominent references to myrrh. The first is when the three Kings brought gifts of gold, frankincense, and myrrh to the infant Jesus soon after his birth. The second is when Mark notes that Jesus was offered wine mixed with myrrh to stop the pain of his crucifixion, but Jesus refused to take it. Finally, the third reference is when John says that Nicodemus brought a seventy-five-pound mixture of myrrh and aloe to anoint the body of Jesus before laying it in the tomb.

Bible verses, such as this one from Song of Solomon, describe the use of myrrh as sensuous incense: "I rose up to open to my beloved; and my hands dropped with myrrh and my fingers with sweet smelling myrrh upon the handles of the lock" (5:5). Psalms (45:8) states: "All thy garments smell of myrrh."

References like those mentioned in the Song of Solomon offer different interpretations to religious and scientific scholars. The former look at these references with devotion, while to the scientist, they describe the aromatic properties of the herb. Some Christian sects still use myrrh for religious ceremonies.

Commiphora gileadensis (Balm of Gilead, Balsam of Gilead)

C. gileadensis, also known as *C. opobalsamum*, was cultivated in the oases of the Dead Sea and surrounding regions of Israel, and the Eastern Mediterranean. Species distribution is now restricted to the hilly and rocky areas around the Red Sea, including Mecca Valley in Saudi Arabia, Yemen, Eritrea, and Ethiopia. It can grow to a height of five metres, and stem diameter can reach 40 centimetres. It bears white to cream coloured flowers. The plant can be propagated through cuttings.

Another name for *C. gileadensis* is the Balm of Gilead or Balsam of Gilead, named after the area near the River Jordan. As Jeremiah 8:22 states, "Is there no balm in Gilead? Is there no physician there? Why then is there no healing for the wound of my people?"

C. gileadensis is believed to be the first plant that the Ethiopian Queen of Sheba brought to Israel. It was highly prized. According to Pliny's *Historia Naturalis*, Rome made large profits from the sale and trade of myrrh from plantations in and around Jericho. In fact, when Romans attacked the Jews of Jerusalem, the latter attempted (unsuccessfully) to destroy the myrrh plantations. Over time, the economic value of myrrh decreased as alternatives arose. Thus, cultivation of the species in the Dead Sea fell dramatically.

Myrrh from the Commiphora genus species is regarded as a cosmetic emollient. Its use in the cosmetic industry today is rare, although Himba women in Namibia still collect and store a mixture of myrrh and fat in cosmetic jars (Nott and Curtis, 2005).

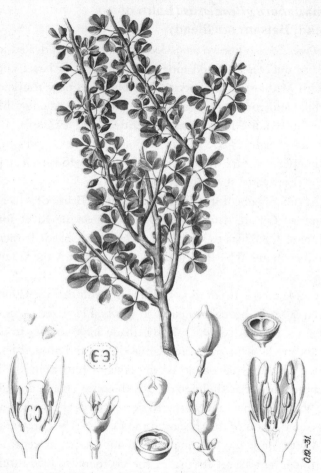

Figure 9 *Commiphora gileadensis* (listed as *Balsamodendron ehrenbergianum*)
by Petronella J.M. Pas, University of Amsterdam

Medicinal uses of Commiphora gileadensis. Hebrew, Greek,
and Roman, followed by Islamic medical texts contain numerous
references to *C. gileadensis*. All parts of the plant, including the
sap, bark, root, leaves, and stem, were regarded as useful through
the first and second centuries AD. The plant was used to treat a

wide range of disorders: headache, stomach ailments, early-stage cataract, impaired vision and hearing, respiratory ailments, and gynecological ailments. It was also used in contraception.

Jews and Romans mixed the sap with old wine or water to make a tonic, which was believed to restore strength, and maintain health. In Unani, the plant was used to treat diseases of the nervous system, especially epilepsy.

Current research has isolated beta caryophyllene from the essential oil of Balsam of Gilead (Amiel et al., 2012). This compound is found in citrus flavours, soaps, skin care products, and so on. Its anti-inflammatory, anaesthetic, antifungal, antiproliferative, and cytotoxic properties have been tested in trials on rats (Iluz, 2010). Studies conducted on albino mice validate the anticonvulsant and neurotoxic properties of the fruit of *C. gileadensis* (Zaidi et al., 2010).

Commiphora myrrha

C. myrrha is a shrub that grows to a height of four metres, and is found in the Arabian Peninsula and in the African regions of Djibouti, Ethiopia, Somalia, and North-eastern Kenya. The tree has a peeling, light-coloured bark with small leaves and small white flowers. As is typical for xerophytes, it has a succulent stem with branches that store water for use during times of stress. The yellowish gum oleoresin is extracted through wounds in the bark. Alpha pinene and limonene compounds give the resin a pine scent. As the resin dries, it turns dark red. The walnut-sized resin bars are collected and distilled to produce myrrh oil. The yield of oil is low, at about 5 to 7 percent.

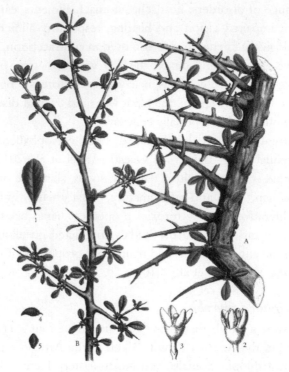

Figure 10 *Commiphora myrrha* by Franz Eugen Köhler

Ancient traders used the Silk Route through Mesopotamia to transport this myrrh to China, by donkey and then by camel, across the entire region from the ports of Petra and Alexandria. Today, the major exporters are Ethiopia, Yemen, and Somalia, although trade data is difficult to obtain because such information is categorised together with other incense-producing plants (e.g., frankincense). *C. myrrha* plantations were produced in Ethiopia using monetary and institutional aid. According to one estimate, new plantations of *C. myrrha* cover more than 170,000 hectares in Ethiopia.

Medicinal uses of Commiphora myrrha. Romans, Egyptians, Greek, and the Chinese used *C. myrrha* as medicine. Written references to myrrh as a perfume and herbal medicine date back to Herodotus in the fifth century BC. Myrrh acts on the mucosa and has antiseptic properties, so Greek and Roman soldiers used it to treat wounds, and sores. In addition to its use as a general tonic and disinfectant, myrrh was also used to treat indigestion, syphilis, and gonorrhoea. It was used as an expectorant to treat respiratory ailments. Because it was believed to promote menstrual flow, it was also used as an abortifacient.

The chemical constituents of myrrh include terpenes, sesquiterpenes, aldehydes, eugenol, resin compounds, volatile and essential oils, and proteins. The presence of sesquiterpenoids indicates neuroprotective properties. In 2011, the European Medicines Agency authorised the use of myrrh tincture to treat minor ulcers and oral inflammation (e.g., gingivitis, stomatitis), minor wounds, and small boils.

In Europe, myrrh is used in nasal decongestants, mouth washes, toothpaste, and other products. The U.S. Food and Drug Administration (FDA) has proposed approving myrrh gum tincture for topical drugs. Studies on mice indicate that myrrh reduces cholesterol and triglycerides, and it increased glucose tolerance in both normal and diabetic rats. Its analgesic properties too were tested in rats (Omer et al., 2011).

China, with a vibrant herbal medicine industry, is a major importer of myrrh, which is known locally as *mo yao*. It is imported in powder and oil forms and used internally and externally to treat rheumatism, circulatory problems, and wounds. It is especially efficacious in treating amenorrhoea, menopause, and uterine tumors (Zhu et al., 2001). As the resin burns slowly, it is also used in aromatherapy.

The European Commission of Health and Consumers Directorate has authorised *C. myrrha* gum extract (also known as myrrh absolute, myrrh oil, gum oil, resin, and resin water) as a perfume, skin and nail conditioner, and masking (odour-preventing) agent in cosmetic and household products. *C. myrrha* leaf extract is also accepted by the Directorate for use in skin care products.

The plant is valued as an ingredient in mouthwashes, toothpaste, creams, and lotions. In the United States, myrrh oleoresin, essential oil, and extracts are approved for use as food additives, and are considered to be in the "Generally Recognised as Safe" category. However, the resin, essential oils, and extracts have not been approved as astringents, or in oral healthcare products.

Bdellium (guggul) from *Commiphora wightii* (Indian Myrrh) and *Commiphora africana*

C. wightii and *C. africana* are believed to be the ingredients of a composite gum called bdellium. Theophrastus was the first to mention bdellium, which he learned about during the campaigns of Alexander the Great in Persia, and India. Dioscorides describes bdellium in *De Materia Medica* as "the tear of an Arabian tree" (i. 80). According to Pliny's *Historia Naturalis* (xii. 35), it is transparent, fragrant, waxy, greasy, and bitter. Pliny mentions elsewhere that the incense from the tree came from Bactria in central Asia.

According to Genesis 2:8–9, bdellium may have been a plant in the Garden of Eden, said to lie in the ancient land of Havilah, which was served by four rivers, and was probably the Euphrates River region in modern Iraq. Others say that references to bdellium in Bible dictionaries indicate that the resin came from *Borassus flabellifer*, which is another xerophyte that grows in India and Arabia, and yields a gum-like fluid called manna.

C. wightii is found in India, where is it called Indian myrrh, and in Eastern Africa, where it is called Guggul. Both *C. wightii* and *C. africana* are sources of bdellium. The thorny shrub is four to six feet tall with yellowish-green papery bark. It inhabits semi-arid to arid regions of Northern India, Central Asia, Northern Africa, Iran, and Iraq. The branches produce a yellow gum that smells like myrrh. The yield of gum is much less than that of *C. gileadensis* or *C. myrrha*. The plant is used locally as incense, and commercially as a perfume binder and food flavouring. Overexploitation has caused rapid deterioration of the species, which, the International Union for Conservation of Nature, has classified as "vulnerable".

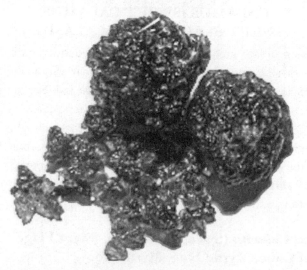

Figure 12 "Commiphora-wightii-resin" by original uploader
Sjschen at en.wikipedia, incense

Medicinal uses of bdellium. The medicinal properties of bdellium are similar to those of *C. myrrha* and *C. gileadensis*. There appears to be consensus on the resin's cholesterol-lowering and analgesic properties. Traditionally, it has been used to treat arthritis, atherosclerosis, skin diseases such as leukoderma, and obesity.

Guggul has been used in Ayurvedic medicine since 600 BC, and there are references to the plant in the *Sushruta Samhita*.

Guggul is used to treat ulcers and sores. Its antibacterial and anthelminthic properties have been studied using the agar well diffusion assay process, and validated. (Pankaj Goel et al, 2010).

According to Ayurveda, Guggul enhances circulation, and helps digestion by producing warmth in the body. Guggulsterone is the major steroid isolated from the plant. Other steroids include diterpenoids, aliphatic esters, carbohydrates, and amino acids.

CALAMUS (SWEET CALAMUS, SWEET FLAG, INDIAN CALAMUS)

Biblical scholars are divided on the true identity of calamus. *Acorus calamus* and Cymbopogon are popular candidates. Both the species are monocots, both prefer moist habitats, and both are sources of aromatic essential oils. Others, such as Benet (1967), have posited a less popular theory that cannabis is the sweet calamus mentioned in the Bible. The name calamus derives from the Hebrew word *qaneh*, which in English translates into "cane." Biblical scholars also interpret "sweet" as an attribute of perfection, and purity.

Acorus Calamus (Sweet Cinnamon, Sweet Flag, Sweet Cane, Myrtle Flag, Myrtle Root)

Calamus is distributed across many parts of the globe, and has many common names: sweet cinnamon, sweet cane, myrtle grass, myrtle flag, and myrtle root. According to the International Union for Conservation of Nature and Natural Resources, the plant is native to India, China, Japan, Korea, South-eastern and Central Asia, Mongolia, Russia, and North America. It grows close to streams, lakes, and other water bodies.

It is a perennial monocot that looks like grass, grows up to two metres tall, and makes a swishing sound in wind. Four varieties are classified by natural polyploidy: diploid, triploid, tetraploid, and hexaploid. The rhizome grows horizontally just below the surface in lengths up to two metres. The blooms are yellowish green, tiny, and inconspicuously attached to the spadix. The leaves and the rhizome are scented. The citrus aroma is strongest in the rhizome, which is whitish pink, and contains the aromatic oil. It has a bitter taste. When the rhizome is dried, it loses 70–75 percent of its weight, but drying enhances the aroma. The rhizome can be stored for up to three years before it loses its aromatic oil.

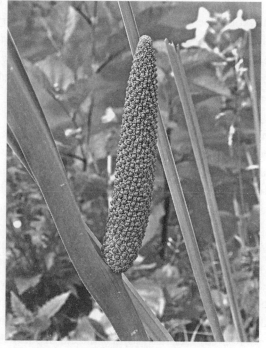

Figure 13 "Acorus calamus1" by H Zell

In ancient times, the plant was probably exported in dried form from Asia to the Mediterranean, where it was used as a substitute for ginger, cinnamon, and nutmeg. Ayurvedic literature, including the *Sushruta Samhita,* lists two species of Acorus in the family Acoraceae as medicinal plants: *A. calamus* and *A. gramineus.*

A. calamus was discovered in the tomb of Pharaoh Tutankhamen of Egypt. Theophrastus in his *Plants IX,* and Pliny in his *Natural History* (25.157) reference an aromatic reed found growing in Lebanon and India, called *Calamus odoratus.* Pliny states that the product from India was superior to that found in the Arabian Peninsula. Dioscorides refers to it as Indian calamus.

Because the use of Holy Anointing Oil was originally exclusive to clergy, it makes sense that the most valuable and expensive ingredients would be sought and imported, if necessary. Verses from the Bible support this claim. For example, Jehovah, through his prophet, reproved the sinful Israelites for "having bought" (in Hebrew, *qani'tha*) no "cane" (*qa·neh'*) for his temple service (Isaiah 43:24).

Also, Jeremiah 6:20 refers to cane received from a "land far away," whereas Ezekiel 27:3, 19 includes cane among the products that the wealthy traded at the port of Tyre, a key Mediterranean port of that time. As Roman culture and then Christianity spread across Europe and beyond, *calamus* was introduced to people across the world. Its linkages with history, culture, and religion added to the mystery of these plants.

A. calamus has been introduced in many European nations; for example, the Tatars introduced it to Poland (fourteenth Century AD). The famous botanist Clusius first cultivated it in Vienna in 1574 from a root obtained from Asia Minor. Leaves were used for thatching roofs, and weaving baskets. From there, it spread to France, Germany, and England around the end of the sixteenth century. Imports to Europe from India and other regions continued until the eighteenth century.

Today, the fragrant oil from the rhizome is used as a flavouring agent in alcoholic beverages, fragrances, perfumes, and sacred oils. According to a 2012 Department of Agriculture and

Agri Food Canada report, the sweet flag oil used by the North American fragrance industry is worth $30 million.

However, this industry diminished greatly after the discovery of carcinogenic chemicals in sweet flag rhizomes. *A. calamus* is still cultivated in parts of India, both as an intercrop with rice, and as a monocrop. Mixed with long pepper and ginger, the aromatic property of the plant is used as a food additive.

The average yield of *A. calamus* rhizomes is estimated as 10–12 metric tons of rhizomes per hectare. Some exports of *A. calamus* rhizome to Singapore and other markets have been reported, mostly for use in herbal medicine. The use of calamus in anointing oil also continues.

Medicinal uses of Acorus calamus. *A. calamus* has been popular among healing traditions around the globe, including Ayurveda, Unani, and Native American medicine. The rhizome, and sometimes the leaves, were used in medicines. For example, travellers routinely carried calamus-based healing oils to treat wounds caused by excessive walking.

When chewed or swallowed fresh, the rhizome is said to stimulate the brain and nervous system, causing euphoria coupled with a calming effect. It can also be dried, ground, pulverised, and converted into capsule form, or mixed into a smoking blend with calamus, tobacco, and other herbs. In Europe, it was common to cover church and mansion floors with *A. calamus* foliage, as the fragrance helped to mask odors caused by poor sanitation, and to deter insects.

The psychedelic properties of the plant are accepted in herbal therapies of Europe, China, and India. In Europe, the rhizome was added to wine and absinthe. In Latin America, it was used as a stimulant, similar to coca leaf. Throughout Europe, it was an ingredient of a hallucinogen called witches' flying ointment. North American tribes like the Sioux held the plant in great esteem. They planted calamus along migration paths and trails. They viewed it as a miracle plant that cured skin diseases, coughs, colds, asthma, and digestive disorders. They also used it in face paint before battle for its stimulating and calming effects. Aromatic garlands were made from the plant, too. Calamus was also extensively used by early American settlers.

The U.S. FDA banned *A. calamus* in 1968, when research indicated that some species of Acorus had carcinogenic chemicals. Research has shown that the North American variety, *A. americanus*, does not have the same carcinogenic chemicals as those found in *A. calamus*. Nevertheless, herbal shops in the United States no longer recommend or dispense products containing this plant.

In 1995, Health Canada listed the species as a "herb used as non-medicinal ingredient in non-prescription drugs for human use." Although the Canadian sub-species does not contain the carcinogenic chemicals, the water of its habitats is often poisoned by hemlock (*Cicuta maculata*).

Cymbopogon citratus (Lemon grass)

C. citratus is a frost-sensitive perennial, with rhizomes and tapering grass-like leaves that grow up 45–60 centimetres long and 10–20 mm wide. It is native to India, Sri Lanka, and the islands of South-eastern Asia. Today, India is the major producer of lemongrass oil, with nearly 80 percent of the total annual production of 600 metric tons. The main buyers are the United States, followed by Japan and Europe. As its use in medicine, food, fragrances, and cosmetics increases, cultivation of the species has expanded to Latin America and the tropical state of Florida in the United States.

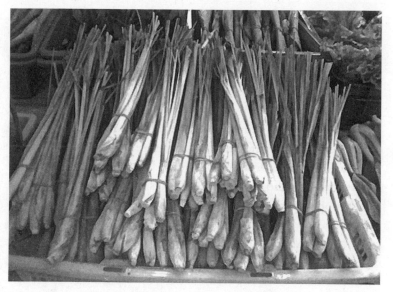

Figure 14 Serai lemongrass, licensed under CC
BY-SA 3.0 via Wikimedia Commons

Biblical scholars, such Zohary (1985), Duke (2010), and Jensen (Danish 2004, English translation 2012), have suggested another species, Cymbopogon, as the true sweet calamus mentioned in the Bible. This species is still found in India, Africa, and Iraq, who exported it to the Mediterranean region during Biblical times. Because Cymbopogon is a skin irritant, it seems an unlikely ingredient in the Holy Anointing Oil.

However, Cymbopogon species are popular spices in Southeastern Asian cuisine, and the grass and essential oil extracts are used in Ayurveda and Traditional Chinese Medicine. Although not used in Roman or Greek cuisine, the essential oil was used in cosmetics and perfumery. It is therefore not inappropriate to consider Cymbopogon as a possible ingredient in the Holy Anointing Oil.

Many references in ancient Greek and Roman literature refer to calamus in ointments, wines, and fragrances. In Pliny the

Elder's *Naturalis Historia* (Book XIII, Chapter 7, Paragraph 9), he mentions a Telinum (fragrant ointment) made of fresh olive oil, cyperus, calamus, yellow melilot, fenugreek, honey, marum, and sweet marjoram. He also mentions an Indian grass with aromatic properties. The comic poet Menander called it the most fashionable perfume. A wine that has a concoction of calamus, costus, spikenard, cinnamon, cardamom, saffron, ginger, and other herbs, is also referred to in literature of that time.

However, the connection between Cymbopogon species, and the calamus mentioned in the Bible, has not yet been established. Many popular spices in Israel, Egypt, Greece, and Rome, up to the fall of the Roman Empire, came from the spice-producing regions of Asia. Adulterating these commodities with low-cost fillers was common. For example, cinnamon was adulterated with cassia, and Arabian frankincense was mixed with that from Ethiopia and India. Thus, perhaps calamus was produced from both *A. calamus* and Cymbopogon species.

Medicinal uses of Cymbopogon citratus. The medicinal properties of lemongrass have been widely studied. It contains 65–85 percent citral and myrcene, which have antibacterial and analgesic properties. It also has restorative, digestive, antitussive, antiviral, analgesic, antiemetic, anticardiopathic, anti-inflammatory (in urinary ducts), diuretic, antispasmodic, diaphoretic, and anti-allergic effects (Negrelle and Gomes, 2007).

Its anti-inflammatory, antimicrobial, antimycobacterial, antiviral, antifungal, antifilarial, antiamoebic, and antimutagenic properties have been studied, and validated in animal trials. The plant is also indicated to possess antipyretic, antiseptic, anticarcinogenic, hypoglycemic, and insecticidal properties. Various active compounds, such as citronel, citronellal, geraniol, terpenes, alcohols, ketones, aldehydes, esters, flavonoids, and phenolic compounds, have been isolated from *C. citratus*, which the U.S. FDA has classified as "Generally Recognised as Safe."

The essential oil is used extensively in the food industry for its fragrance, and its positive impact on the digestive system, because it helps reduce flatulence, colic, and stomach cramps, in addition to being carminative, and astringent. The herb is also a traditional Brazilian medicine, and is believed to help calm the mind, and to treat muscular spasms, cramps, and fatigue.

C. citratus grass has been used by the Brazilian Quilombolas tribe as an anxiolytic to decrease blood pressure, and calm individuals. The oil is applied externally to aid muscle tone, tissue tension, headaches, arthritis pain, and acne. It has a positive impact on the parasympathetic nervous system by reducing nervous system stress, and correcting poor circulation.

In Ayurveda, it is used to provide relief in cases of respiratory distress, cough, sore throat, laryngitis, and fever. It is useful in preventing colitis, indigestion, and other gastroenteritis ailments. According to the principles of Traditional Chinese Medicine, Cymbopogon, or *xiang mao*, has acrid and warm properties, and is used to treat headaches, abdominal pain, and rheumatic pain.

Other uses of Cymbopogon citratus. Lemongrass oil is extracted by steam distillation, which separates the oil from the water. The pleasant lemony flavour makes it a popular ingredient in skin care products, cosmetics, soaps, and perfumes. Mixed with virgin coconut oil, it is called Oil of Negros, and is used in aromatherapy. A by-product of extraction is a scented water that is used in skin care products such as lotions, creams, and toners.

The essential oils of *Cymbopogon* species are used in beverages, foodstuffs, fragrances, household products, personal care products, pharmaceuticals, and in tobacco. Lemongrass is extensively used to flavour soups, salads, and curries in South-eastern Asia, China, and the Caribbean. It is rich in vitamins and minerals, and is a preferred ingredient in Thai food. It is used to spice pickles and marinades, and is often paired with garlic, ginger, and cilantro. In Brazil, a tea infused with *C. citratus* extract is prepared from fresh or dry leaves.

Cymbopogon martinii (Palmarosa Grass, Rosha Grass, Indian Geranium)

Cymbopogon martinii looks similar to lemongrass. It is a tall grass (1.8 to 2.4 metres), found in wild areas of Southern Asia, the Middle East, Africa, Australia, and Latin America. It is widely cultivated for its essential oil. The oil was imported from India to Constantinople (modern day Istanbul,) and Europe, until the eighteenth century for use in soaps and perfumes.

Prior to the 1990s, India was the only producer and exporter of palmarosa oil, which is reduced by steam distilling the aromatic grass, and is more than 80 percent pure. Essential oil yields vary from 1 to 1.5 percent. As production of palmarosa improved in Brazil, Guatemala, and Colombia, the quality of oil produced in these areas surpassed that of Indian palmarosa. Synthetic substitutes have also adversely affected production. Today, the major importers of palmarosa oil are the United States, Europe, and Australia.

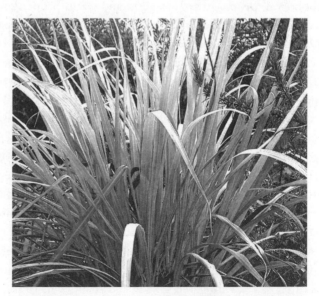

Figure 15 "Cymbopogon martini" by Alabama Essential Oils

The two major varieties of this species are *C. martinii var motia* and *C. martinii var sofia*. Both yield palmarosa oil (motia oil, and sofia oil, respectively). Though similar, motia oil is the preferred variety. Sofia oil is also called ginger grass oil. The essential oil is fragrant and smells like roses, so it is sometimes used as an adulterant in more expensive rose oil. The oil is pale yellow to yellowish green in colour, and has a thin consistency. It blends well with geranium, bergamot, rosemary, lime, and ylang-ylang oil.

Harvesting for manufacturing essential oil should be done within seven to ten days after the flowers open, with the best oil yields from fully open flowers. The grass is cut about six inches above the ground, and harvested four times per year. The highest oil yields are achieved in the first four years, at which point it is normally recommended to replant the grass. The harvested grass is dried in the field for a few days, and then stored in shade to reduce its weight by half. This makes distillation and transportation more efficient.

Medicinal uses of Cymbopogon martinii. Ayurvedic healers have used this grass to treat respiratory (e.g., cough, cold, bronchitis, asthma) and digestive disorders (e.g., flatulence, dyspepsia). The species is regarded to possess neuroprotective properties, so it is used to treat depression, and other neurological disorders. It is also regarded as a general immunostimulant for the endocrine system, uterus, and heart.

In aromatherapy, the oil is believed to uplift the mood, reduce stress, soothe the nerves, and create a sense of well-being. *C. martinii* is a powerful antioxidant. The essential oil is used in Chinese aromatherapy to treat inflammation that causes chronic pain, rheumatism, and indigestion. Its antimicrobial, antifungal, antiviral, and antibacterial properties have been demonstrated in animal trials (Lawrence et al., 2012).

The essential oil of *C. martinii* is used in perfumes, soaps, shampoos, tobacco, fragrances, and massage and bath oils.

Additionally, several mosquito repellents are manufactured using palmarosa oil because of its effectiveness against malaria-causing mosquitoes.

CINNAMON

Cinnamon is one of the more famous spices from Biblical and pre-Biblical times. It originates from a number of species, including *Cinnamomum zeylanicum syn* in the Family Lauraceae. *Cinnamomum brumannii, Cinnamomum cassia,* and *Cinnamomum loureirii, classified as cassias,* grow in Indonesia, China, and Vietnam, respectively.

Cinnamon and cassia have similar aromatic properties, but they differ in flavour, eugenol content, and look and texture of the bark. Cinnamon is milder, with less eugenol and a thinner, light-coloured bark. Cinnamon is more expensive, compared to cassia.

Cinnamomum verum yields the most valuable cinnamon, known as true cinnamon. Cinnamon is also produced from the aromatic bark of an unrelated species belonging to a different genus and family, *Canella winterana,* from the Canellaceae family. According to a 2012 FAO statistic, 186,000 hectares of land is used to cultivate Cinnamomum and *C. winterana.*

Total annual production in China, Indonesia, Sri Lanka, and Vietnam is estimated to be 155,000 metric tons, which accounts for 98 percent of the world's supply. Indonesian cinnamon comprises two-thirds of the global production, with the rest from India, Vietnam, and China.

Cinnamon and cassia were immensely valuable, and cinnamon in particular was prized in the Mediterranean. Both spices were given as gifts to gods and emperors. An inscription records such a gift to the temple of Apollo at Miletus in Thebes, which dates back to the early seventh century BC. Pliny states that a pound of cassia or cinnamon could cost up to 10 months'of a labourer' wages. Later, Roman Emperor Nero burnt a year's worth of cinnamon and myrrh for the funeral of his wife.

The Bible contains four references to cinnamon: three times in the Old Testament, and once in the New Testament. Song of Songs, for example, states: "A garden locked is my sister, my bride, a garden locked, a fountain sealed. Your channel is an orchard of pomegranates with all choice fruits, henna with nard, nard and saffron, calamus and cinnamon, with all trees of frankincense, myrrh and aloes, with all chief spices—a garden fountain, a well of living water, and flowing streams from Lebanon" (Song of Songs 4:12–15).

Proverbs describes using spices like cinnamon in romantic allurement. Cinnamon is also described as one of the finest spices in Exodus 30:23. Revelations 18:11–13 describes the devaluation of spices, and other valuable goods during the fall of Rome, and destruction of the Jewish temple at Jerusalem, during the first millennium.

Exodus 32:23–24 distinguishes between cinnamon and cassia. Cinnamon was more expensive, and its aroma was regarded as superior to cassia. Cassia was often used as an adulterant of cinnamon. The recipe for Holy Anointing Oil calls for twice as much cinnamon as cassia. Although this distinction is blurred today, as both spices are called cinnamon, true cinnamon is still valued higher than cassia. Cinnamon is used extensively all over the world in cuisine, confections, cosmetics, soaps, and incense.

The inner bark yields 0.5–1 percent aromatic essential oil, depending on the species. It is used as a seasoning in food, such as meat and baked goods, and in drinks, such as coffee. It is also an appetite suppressant.

Cinnamon contains the alkaloid coumarin, a fragrant chemical used in cosmetics, colognes, and tobacco. Sri Lankan and Indonesian cinnamons have lower levels of alkaloid. When consumed regularly, coumarin is believed to impact the liver negatively.

Germany's Federal Institute for Risk Assessment issued a warning that a 132-pound adult who regularly eats more than 2 grams (0.07 ounces) of cassia cinnamon daily could suffer harmful side effects. The agency reports no side effects, however, from occasional consumption of cinnamon. Other European countries have issued formal warnings advising consumers accordingly. The U.S. FDA lists cassia and Ceylon cinnamon as safe for human consumption, but it does not specify quantities.

Cinnamomum zeylanicum Syn C. Verum (True Cinnamon, Sri Lankan Cinnamon)

Cinnamomum zeylanicum syn C. verum is one of the most prized cinnamons. It comes from the inner bark of the tree, which grows in the tropical evergreen forests of Sri Lanka and parts of Southern India, mainly Western Ghats. The tree grows to a height of 10–15 metres and can reach 30 centimetres in diametre. True cinnamon trees have a thinner and lighter coloured bark. The taste of Sri Lankan cinnamon is lighter, with citrus overtones. The estimated production of *C. verum* cinnamon from Sri Lanka is 10,000 metric tons, about 90 percent of the world supply.

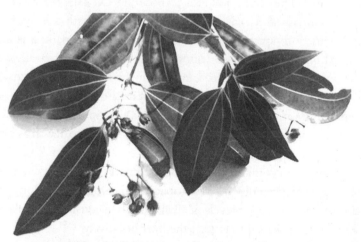

Figure 16 "Cinnamomum verum1," licensed under Public Domain via Wikimedia Commons

In ancient times, Sri Lankan cinnamon was the most prized spice, and it continues to attract premium prices. When the Portuguese occupied the Kandy region of Sri Lanka in 1518, they enslaved the local population and monopolised the Sri Lanka cinnamon trade. The Dutch displaced the Portuguese in 1638 and controlled the trade for another 150 years, until the British defeated the Dutch in 1784. By then, cinnamon cultivation had expanded to other parts of the world, and its price fell.

Today, the species is cultivated in many parts of the world. It is an invasive species in Madagascar, the Seychelles, and other tropical Pacific islands, Brazil, Colombia, Mexico, and a few countries in Eastern Africa. The plant is coppiced every two years, to enhance shoot growth and yield.

When the tree is 3–4 years old, the outer woody bark is stripped of the shoots and discarded, and the supple inner bark is removed in long strips. This operation is best done during the rainy season when peeling the bark is relatively easy. As these peelings dry, they curl up in the form of long sticks, which are then cut into 5–10 cm segments called quills.

The chemical composition of the quills includes cinnamaldehyde, gums, tannin, mannitol, coumarin, calcium oxalate, aldehyde, eugenol, pinene, and minerals. Sri Lankan cinnamon is easily ground into a powder, whereas the tough and woody texture of other species can damage the grinder. Once ground, however, it is difficult to distinguish the origin of the cinnamon.

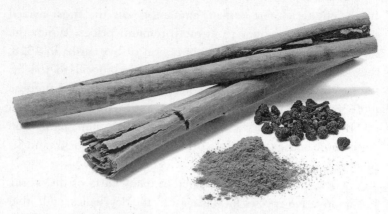

Figure 17 "Cinnamomum verum spices" by Simon A. Eugster, own work, licensed under CC BY-SA 3.0 via Wikimedia Commons

Three essential oils are extracted from cinnamon trees: eugenol from the leaves, cinnamaldehyde from the bark, and camphor from the root. Leaf oil yield is 0.7–1.2 percent, and the eugenol is used to synthesise vanillin, and converted into iso-eugenol for use as a flavouring in confections. Because of its warm, spicy, and harsh odor, this oil is also used in soaps, perfumes, and insecticides. Bark oil is extracted by steam distilling bark, twigs, and chips. The essential oil content in the bark varies from 0.5–2 percent.

The oleoresin contains volatile oil, fixed oil, and other extracts, and is used to flavour food and soft drinks, as well as dental, and pharmaceutical preparations. It is less popular in perfumes, because it is a skin irritant. Its aroma, which is rich in cinnamaldehyde, is delicate, sweet, and pungent.

The seeds contain about 30 percent fixed oil, obtained by crushing and boiling the ripe fruit. This oil is used in India for candle making. A gum or resin is also extracted from the bark with the help of organic solvents. A cheaper alternative to cinnamon leaf oil is clove leaf oil.

Medicinal uses of Cinnamomum zeylanicum syn C. verum.
The medicinal properties of cinnamon have been scientifically studied, and preliminary results suggest it has antidiabetic properties (Ranasinghe et al., 2012). Other studies indicate that cinnamon can reduce cholesterol, thus making the species cardio-protective (Shan et al., 2007).

It is used as a tonic and sedative in childbirth. When applied to the skin, cinnamon oil causes blood to rush to the applied area, which helps nourish the skin and produces a tingling sensation. It also produces a temporary plump look that minimises wrinkles and lines, especially around the eyes. Applying oil with a few drops of cinnamon essential oil helps relieve itchy scalp and acne.

The bark has astringent, antiseptic, antifungal, carminative, antioxidant, antimicrobial, and stimulant properties. It is used as a remedy against colds and digestive ailments like diarrhoea and colic. In European phytomedicine, cinnamon bark oil (0.05–0.2 g daily intake) is used in teas and other galenicals for appetite loss, and dyspeptic disturbances. The maximum permitted level in food products is 0.06 percent.

CASSIA

Cassia differs from cinnamon in strength, and quality. The bark and quills are darker, coarser, and woodier, and the bark is reddish brown. Cassia is sweet and spicy like cinnamon, but more pungent. Its buds are like cloves but with a slight aroma. Nowadays, true cinnamon and cassia are colloquially referred to as cinnamon, and most cinnamon sold in the market today is cassia. It is exported across the globe from Indonesia, Vietnam, China, and India.

The main species yielding cassia are *Cinnamomum burmannii*, *Cinnamomum aromaticum syn, Cinnamomum loureirei*, and *Cinnamomum cassia*. A limited amount of cassia is also produced in India from *Cinnamomum tamala*.

Cassia is part of the Chinese five-spice powder with Sichuan pepper, cloves, fennel, star anise, and cloves. A popular sauce in Chinese food, known as the "master sauce," contains a five-spice powder with liquorice. Similarly, cassia is an ingredient in the Indian masala that is used in nearly every Indian curry. Cassia is also used in baked goods, drinks, and cuisine, across the globe.

There are references to cassia in the Ebers papyrus. Rufus of Ephesus (c. 50 AD) mentions cassia as one the ingredients in the Egyptian incense Kyphi, but other documented recipes by scholars such as Dioscorides mention cardamom. Pliny mentions the use of cassia as a flavouring agent in wines (nat. 14, 107f). The third-century BC Greek scholar Theophrastus described megaleion, a poultice of burnt resin, cassia, cinnamon, oil of balanos, and myrrh, that helped relieve wound inflammation. Sappho was the first Greek to reference cassia in a poem (c. seventh century BC).

The Jews used cassia as incense in the First and Second Temples of Jerusalem. It was one of the 11 ingredients in the concentrated Jewish incense, Ketoret, which was used to prepare the Jewish temple for worship. The Bible mentions cassia several times as an ingredient of the Holy Anointing Oil. Ezekiel 27:19 and Psalm 45:8 reveal the existence of trade in spices, including cassia and cinnamon, which were used in unguents to perfume hair and garments in Greek and Roman times.

When the Romans acquired global power (c. 200 BC), the Mediterranean ports began receiving large quantities of imported spices, and other products from India, Malacca (Maluku) Islands, and the Arabian Peninsula. Goods traveled from the ports of Alexandria and Tyre to Africa, Europe, and Asia.

Literature surveys indicate that the major sources of cassia were Indonesia and India. The majority of trade was by boat via the Indian Ocean and the Red Sea, although the Silk Route from

China was also used to trade with Mesopotamia. In China, cassia is called *kwei* and is referenced in Traditional Chinese Medicine dating back to Sheng Nung (c. 2700 BC).

The species is mentioned extensively in Ayurveda. It is also an important culinary spice in India and Eastern Asia. Cassia is also used extensively in the cosmetic industry. In grated and essential oil forms, the product is mixed with olive oil or petroleum jelly to produce skin treatment products. As in most traditional medicine practices, cassia is often administered in combination with other herbs. Thus, conclusive evidence of its medicinal impact is difficult to obtain.

Cinnamomum burmannii
(Indonesian Cassia or Padang Cassia)

Cinnamomum burmannii grows in the wet evergreen forests of Indonesia, Malaysia, and the Philippines. It yields a cheaper variety of cinnamon, popularly called Indonesian cassia. This shrub reaches a height of about seven metres and is harvested at five years of age. In crops, it can survive for about 20 years, and probably lives longer in the wild.

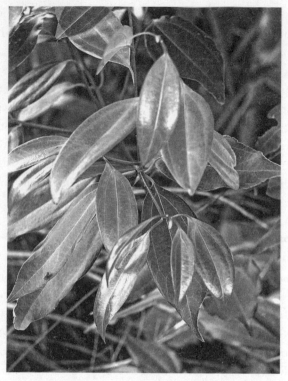

Figure 18 "Starr 090213-2452 Cinnamomum burmannii" by Forest & Kim Starr, licensed under CC by 3.0 via Wikimedia Commons

The bark and leaves are used in cuisine, processed food, confections, and drinks. The bark is sold in quills, and the quill of Indonesian cassia has a single and thicker layer compared to true cinnamon. Cassia is quite popular in the United States, where it is used extensively in commercial baking. It is cheaper than Chinese cassia (*C. cassia*) but lacks depth of aroma.

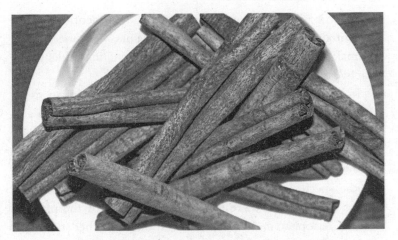

Figure 19 "Cinnamon Quills" by Jonathunder, own work

The chemical constituents of *C. burmannii* are similar to other cassias and include cinnamyl alcohol, coumarin, cinnamic acid, cinnamaldehyde, anthocynin, and essential oils together with constituents of sugar, protein, crude fats, pectin, and others. Coumarin, as previously mentioned, is toxic to humans when ingested regularly. Prolonged use can cause liver inflammation, and jaundice. The maximum recommended daily intake of coumarin is 0.1 mg per kilogram of body weight, and 1 teaspoon of cassia powder contains between 6–12 mg coumarin. Thus, the European Food Safety Authority limits the quantity of cassia that can be safely ingested.

Medical uses of Cinnamomum burmannii. The medicinal properties of *C. burmannii* are similar to those of other cassia species. Studies show that the leaf contains 0.4 percent essential oil, consisting of cinnamaldehyde (45–62 percent) and eugenol (10 percent). The leaf is also rich in monoterpenes and sesquiterpenes.

The plant has been shown to possess analgesic, anti-inflammatory, anticoagulant, antibacterial, antifungal, antidiabetic, antitumor, antithrombotic, and antirheumatic properties. The powdered bark is traditionally used for the treatment of nausea, flatulent dyspepsia, coughs, chest complaints, diarrhoea, gripe, and malaria. Studies have indicated that trans-cinnamaldehyde is its active anti-inflammatory component.

In animal studies, Indonesian cassia has been shown to be effective against a range of bacteria, such as *Escherichia coli* and *Staphylococcus aureus*. Similar studies have found anti-inflammatory, analgesic, and antidiabetic properties. Chewing gums containing Indonesian cassia were found to possess antibacterial properties, and the species is used to treat dental caries and periodontitis. Studies indicate that there is a prospect of use of the plant in treating nasopharyngeal carcinoma, though further trials are needed.

Cinnamomum Aromaticum Syn Cinnamomum Cassia (Chinese Cinnamon)

Cinnamomum aromaticum syn cinnamomum cassia is an evergreen tree that originated in tropical regions of Southern China, and has also been found in India, Vietnam, and neighbouring Asian countries. It grows to a height of 10–12 metres. The bark and buds are used as a spice.

Cassia essential oil, produced from *C. cassia,* is distilled from the bark, twigs, and leaves, whereas true cinnamon oil is distilled from the inner bark only. Compared to Sri Lankan and Indonesian cinnamon, the flavour of *C. cassia* bark is much stronger, because of its higher essential oil content. Chinese cassia is therefore more expensive, sometimes three times the price of its counterparts. Similarly, cinnamon oil can be five times costlier than cassia oil.

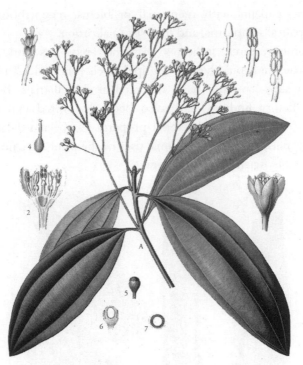

Figure 20 *Cinnamomum aromaticum* by Franz Eugen Köhler

Medicinal uses of Cinnamomum aromaticum syn cinnamomum cassia. The bark and leaves of *C. aromaticum syn cinnamomum cassia* are used as medicine. Traditionally, this plant is used to treat a range of common gastrointestinal ailments like flatulence, dyspepsia, stomachache, nausea, diarrhoea, cramps, and loss of appetite. The species is believed to purify the blood, and assuage disorders caused by high blood pressure.

The bark is useful in treating cold, cough, bronchitis, chest pain, and respiratory ailments. Bark oil contains cinnamaldehyde, phenol, coumarin, benzaldehyde, chavicol, aromatic aldehyde, isoeugenol, and other aromatic aldehydes. The plant is also used to treat patients with menstrual problems, menorrhoea, and menopausal symptoms, and to assist in abortion.

Some research indicates that the spice has antidiabetic properties and could help lower lipid levels (Liu et al., 2014), but these claims have not been validated in clinical trials. Besides, contradictory findings have also been discovered (Yu et al., 2010). The plant's antibacterial property has been validated in animal trials, but most traditional uses of the plant have not been validated by scientific experiments.

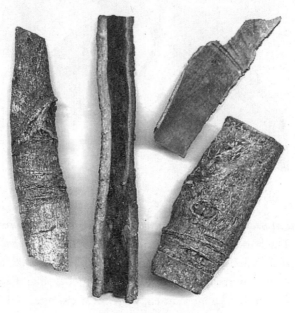

Figure 21 "Cassia bark" licensed under CC BY-SA 3.0 via Wikimedia Commons

C. aromaticum syn cinnamomum cassia is among the top 50 medicinal plants in Traditional Chinese Medicine. It is used to treat colds, flatulence, nausea, diarrhoea, and painful menstrual periods. It improves qi, or human vitality. It is considered useful for people who feel hot in their body but have cold feet.

The pungent bark and sweet flavour are believed to help the yang (life) in the heart, liver, spleen, and kidney. In combination with other herbs like ginger and aconite, cassia helps to treat a range of diseases, from the common cold, to impotence. In Ayurveda, a drop or two of essential oil in a vaporiser or burner during *Pranayama*, or Yogic breathing exercises, helps reduce depression and brings overall calmness to the mind.

Cinnamomum loureirii
(Vietnamese Cassia, Saigon Cassia)

Cinnamomum loureirii is another of the cassia-yielding species in the wet evergreen forest regions of Vietnam, and neighbouring countries. Among *C. verum* (true cinnamon), *C. cassia*, and *C. loureirii*, *C. loureirii* has the most intense flavour, with the highest quantity of essential oil at 1–5 percent and 25 percent cinnamaldehyde content. Thus, it is the most expensive of the cassias that are marketed as cinnamon today.

Like Chinese cassia (*C. cassia*), Vietnamese cassia has only small quantities of eugenol, which gives it a clove-like aroma. Whole buds are used as a food spice, and *C. loureirii* is highly valued in China and Japan for its strong flavour. *C. loureirii* is commonly used in Traditional Chinese Medicine, and other herbal practices.

Exports of *C. loureirii* ceased for more than 20 years during the Vietnam War. After the war, exploitation of the species for cassia production began again. It is now exported to North American and other global markets. U.S. spice importers also buy it in rough bark form, and market it in America as "whole cinnamon." Bark of this cassia is harvested when the trees reach 10–12 years of age, which is much older than the harvesting age for other cassia species. Additionally, the branches are stripped of their bark, unlike the coppicing and shoot-stripping techniques for other species.

Multiple species of Cinnamomum genus yield cassia, including *C. cassia*, *C. burmannii*, and *C. loureirii*. True cinnamon comes from

C. verum syn C zeylanicum. In trade, both cinnamon and cassia are loosely referred to as cinnamon, although there are differences in flavour, and molecular composition.

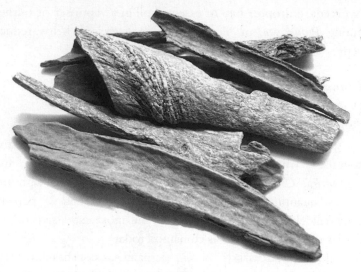

Figure 22 "Saigon cinnamon" by Badagnani, own work, licensed under CC BY 3.0 via Wikimedia Commons

CHAPTER 3

HERBS IN ANCIENT INCENSES AND PERFUMES

∽

Plants have been in use since time immemorial for their scent. Incense, a material derived from plants that emits an aroma when burned, has had many uses throughout history. Nearly every religion throughout the world has used incense in religious or spiritual rituals to propitiate gods, raise spirits, and purify souls. Incense also cleans and freshens temples and homes. Additionally, it has been used in offerings to royalty, perfumes, food, and drink.

According to Wikipedia, the earliest use of incense was during the fifth Dynasty of Egypt (c. 2345–2494 BC). However, the Indus Valley people and the Sumerians likely also used incense. Flowers with aromatic scents like marigold, jasmine, and *mahua* were included in temple offerings and secular and religious events in Hinduism, Buddhism, Taoism, and other Eastern religions.

The oldest Veda, *Rig Veda*, mentions the use of incense in the *Yagnya* fire ritual. In ancient Hindu tradition, knowledge passed from generation to generation orally; thus, based on extant practices, it is probable that the holy fire was scented with locally available aromatic wood and materials like pine, sandalwood, camphor, and cinnamon.

Many of these incenses were imported from Africa, the Arabian Peninsula, India, the Malacca Islands, and China via the trade routes. Others were grown and cultivated locally. Even today, throughout India, it is common to adorn houses, temples, and other places with flowers, leaves, and branches, on special occasions.

Greece, Rome, and Egypt also used incense in religious worship, daily life, celebrations, and medicine. There are multiple references to frankincense, myrrh, cedar, cinnamon, cloves, balsam, aloes, pine, myrtle, benzoin, labdanum, mastic, juniper berry, cardamom, and calamus, in religious and secular literature of the ancient Greeks and Egyptians.

Many of these herbs were also ingredients in Kyphi, the incense used in Egyptian temples and homes, indicating the cultural influence of the Egyptians on the Jews, and other peoples under pharaonic control. Fragrant ointments were applied to clothing, as well as the body and hair. Incense was used in the temples of ancient Egyptian gods Ra and Horus.

Pliny the Elder recorded that alabaster containers were the preferred means of storing raw incense resins, which seems to be accurate, because 350 litters of resins stored in alabaster containers were found in the tomb of King Tut (c. 1342 BC) in 1922. The resins were still active and viable.

Unlike perfumes today, however, the perfumes of antiquity were oily ointments, dense pomades, and balsams (syrupy mixtures of tars and etheric oils). The favourite scents of the ancient Mediterranean were those of rose, lily, iris, sage, thyme, marjoram, saffron, mint, and anise. Frankincense, myrrh, and lavender were regularly used in religious rites. They were burned, releasing a fragrant smoke into the surrounding atmosphere.

The Bible, the Quran, and *the Hadiths* also contain numerous references to the use of incense. The traditional use of incense for worship ebbed with the rise of Christianity, but its value in the pre-Christian era continued until the birth of Christ, and for centuries afterward. Spices were valuable commodities. Pliny wrote in the first century AD that the Arabians were the richest people in the world because of their profits from the spice trade. The Three Kings who visited Baby Jesus at the time of his birth brought gifts of gold, frankincense, and myrrh. There are also multiple references to the use of various herbs and spices to perfume clothes, to commemorate burials, and to express love, romance, and joy.

There are twenty-one references to incense burning in the Bible, including Luke 1:8–11, Hebrews 9:1–4, and Revelation 5:6–8. Incense was also used in the embalming of Jesus' body. Initially, the early Christians forbade the use of incense in churches. Today, the Eastern Orthodox, Lutheran, and Roman Catholic churches continue to use incense for religious purposes.

Incense was a symbol of prayer for the Jews. In Psalm 141:2, David says, "Let my prayer be counted as incense before you, and the lifting up of my hands as the evening sacrifice!" The Talmud records an ancient tradition, perhaps dating back to the second Temple of Jerusalem (c. 516 BC), of mixing 11 ingredients to produce Ketoret for use in the Jewish temples of Jerusalem. The incense comprised "balm, onycha, galbanum and frankincense, each in the quantity of seventy manehs; of myrrh, cassia, spikenard and saffron, each sixteen manehs by weight; of costus twelve, of aromatic rind three, and of cinnamon nine manehs; of lye obtained from leek nine kabs; of salt the Sodom the fourth of a kab, and of the smoke raiser (a herb that makes the smoke of the incense rise) a minute quantity" (Rabbi Louis Jacob, *My Jewish Learning*). It was burned twice daily in the Holy Temple and helped mask the odour from the animal sacrifices.

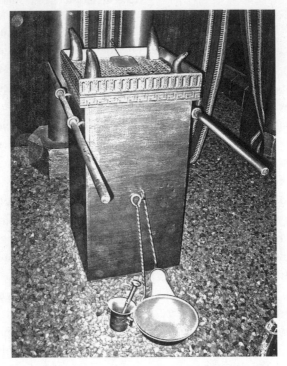

Figure 23 "Timna Tabernacle Incense altar" by Ori229, own work, licensed under CC BY-SA 3.0 via Wikimedia Commons

This chapter describes the principal plants (and one animal) referenced in *the Bible*, as components of incense and perfume: agarwood, frankincense, stacte, styrax, benzoin, galbanum, spikenard, saffron, onycha, operculum, costus, and henna.

AGARWOOD (AQUILARIA SPECIES: ALOES, ALOESWOOD, *OUDH*)

Botanically, the tropical evergreen species of agarwood belongs to the genus Aquilaria, and family Thymelaceae. Agarwood perfume can be extracted from eight species belonging to this genus. The four principal species are *Aquilaria sinensis*, *Aquilaria malaccensis*, *Aquilaria agallocha*, and *Aquilariacrassna*.

Agarwood, or aloeswood, is often confused with aloe vera, which is a purgative. However, aloe vera has no fragrance, which likely eliminates it as a source of agarwood. The following verse perhaps led to this confusion: "How beautiful are your tents, Jacob, your dwelling places, Israel! Like valleys they spread out, like gardens beside a river, like aloes planted by the Lord, like cedars beside the waters" (Numbers 24:5–6). This verse suggests that aloes was local to Israel, but *A. malaccensis* and other aloes-yielding plants are native to Southern Asia.

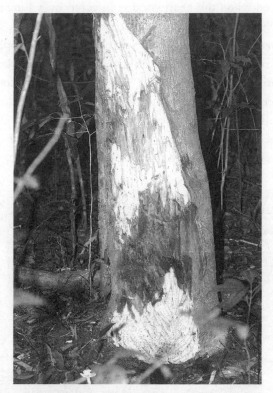

Figure 24 "Aquilaria crassna" by I. Blaise Droz, licensed under
CC BY-SA 3.0 via Wikimedia Commons

A. sinensis is the smallest of the four species, at just 5–15 metres in height. *A. malaccensis* and *A. agallocha* can grow to a height of 15 to 40 metres. The flowers of the tree emanate fragrance at night only. *A. malaccensis* and *A. agallocha* are found in Eastern India, Bangladesh, and Myanmar. Other species extend across Southeastern Asia in Malaysia, Indonesia, Thailand, Cambodia, Vietnam, and the Philippines.

Trees older than 60 years are best for extracting resin. Dark wood without white streaks indicates the presence of resin, which is produced when the heartwood is infected by a fungus. These fungi include Aspergillus spp., Botryodyplodia spp., Diplodia spp., Fusarium spp, Penicillium spp., and Pythium spp. (Anon., 1998a; Santoso, 1996, cited in Soehartono and Mardiastuti, 1997; Wiriadinata, 1995). As the wood rots, it produces a resin. This process can take centuries, making agarwood resin a scarce resource. Furthermore, in nature, the fungi infect only seven percent of the trees. Thus, the use of agarwood as timber is limited. However, extraction of resin requires the tree to be logged.

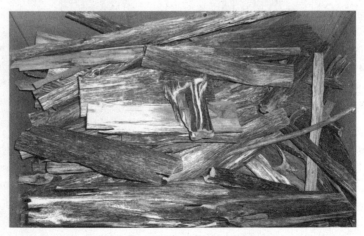

Figure 25 "Agarwood" by Hafizmuar at Wikipedia, licensed under
CC BY-SA 3.0 via Wikimedia Commons

High demand for the resin has led to overexploitation. The tree is not conducive to agroforestry cultivation either, as slow growth and low infection rates have reduced the return of investment substantially. The International Union for Conservation of Nature classified it as vulnerable, and the Convention on International Trade in Endangered Species of Wild Fauna and Flora placed it in Appendix II. Appendix II species trade is constrained to protect their numbers to be so depleted that they are likely to go extinct. Additionally, India and Bhutan have restricted extraction to dead and fallen trees only. This international regulation has helped to control demand and protect these trees for future generations, though the oleoresin that is locally produced from these forests is more likely to be illegally procured.

With just seven percent of the tree crop infected with the necessary fungi, forestry experts have tried to inoculate the fungus artificially by inflicting deep blazes (cuts) or bores in the trunks of young trees and injecting the fungus directly into the heartwood. With this method, oleoresin can be extracted from the stem and branches of trees that are younger than 10 years old. This method has been successful in some of the smaller agarwood species, like *A. sinensis*.

Extensive plantations of *A. sinensis* exist in tropical regions of China, such as Hainan, Guangdong, and Hunan, as well as Vietnam, Thailand, Malaysia, Indonesia, and Cambodia. However the quality of oleoresin from these plantations is not as good as that found in nature. This further explains the huge price variations in the market.

In ancient times, agarwood was popular in Rome, Greece, Arabia, Persia, Egypt, India, and China. It was used in embalming (e.g., John 19:39–40), and such use continues in some Middle Eastern areas, such as Yemen. Historical records show that *A. sinensis* trees grew abundantly in Dongguan City (now Guangdong Province, China) about 400 years ago. Paper was made from its bark and used in Eastern India, and in China. The incense remains popular in many regions today, where it is used in pharmaceutical, personal care, and household products.

Like cinnamon, pepper, and other spices, aloes was imported from India in a vibrant trade that dates back to at least 3000 BC. Pure agarwood is heavy and sinks in water, and literature shows that the Chinese imported *ch'enhsiang* (the incense that sinks) from Vietnam during the Han Dynasty (200 BC–220 AD).

Ancient medical Sanskrit texts refer to *anarya*, indicating that the tree was found in areas not inhabited by the Aryan people. (The Aryans often referred to local indigenous people living in the regions they occupied as anarya, which was also a derogatory term used to describe people who did not follow the cultural codes of the ruling Aryan people). Agarwood or aloeswood was probably imported from the eastern tribal regions of India into the Indo-Gangetic plains, where the Aryan population was concentrated.

Hoardes of aloeswood, muslin, and pepper were recovered when the Byzantine King Heraclius (611–641 AD) sacked the imperial residence of the King of Persia. Arabic and Persian writings from 1100 AD and later contain multiple references to it. The cuneiform tablets from the Mesopotamian region also reference aloeswood.

Ancient Islamic texts contain numerous references to agarwood, or *oudh*. Archaeological evidence reveals that oudh was exported from India and Indonesia, largely in the form of oil and wood products. The Hadiths describe it as a treatment for throat-related ailments, as in the following text:

> Umm Qais, daughter of Mihsan, the sister of 'Ukasha b. Mihsan said: I visited Allah's Messenger along with my son who had not, by that time, been weaned and he urinated over his (clothes). He ordered water to be brought and sprinkled (it) over them. She (further) said: I

visited him (Allah's Apostle) along with my son and I had squeezed the swelling in the uvula, whereupon he said: Why do you afflict your children by compressing like this? Use this Indian aloeswood, for it contains seven types of remedies, one among them being a remedy for pleurisy. It is applied through the nose for a swelling of the uvula and poured into the side of the mouth for pleurisy. (Book 26 of Sahih Muslim, #5487)

Today, the Middle East is the largest consumer of agarwood products. The oil is a principal ingredient in 400 fragrances. Oudh wood chips are used in rosary beads and necklaces, incense, powders, and green tea. Incense is used to perfume clothes before prayer, and wood chips are burned to welcome and honor guests. Efforts to create a synthetic substitute for oudh have been unsuccessful. Thus, authentic oudh continues to attract high prices and high demand.

The United Arab Emirates often serves as a distribution centre between the Middle East, India, Indonesia, Malaysia, Hong Kong, Singapore, Taiwan, Vietnam, and Cambodia. One Saudi Arabian agarwood retailer has more than 500 specialty retail stores in 17 countries, with a customer base of 600,000. This retailer imports five metric tonnes of unprocessed agarwood annually.

The trade volume of unprocessed agarwood has been estimated at 6,843 metric tonnes for 1993–2003 in Taiwan (www.gaharuonline.com, quoting TRAFFIC, a wildlife non-government organisation recognised by the International Union for Conservation of Nature, and Convention on International Trade in Endangered Species of Wild Fauna and Flora sources). Much of this wood, which varies in price from US $3,000 to $30,000 per kilogram, is used for Chinese medicine. Other uses, such as in high-quality ornamental sculptures, can go up to $100,000 per kilogram.

In Japan and Korea, incense sticks are made from agarwood. Processed oil prices range from $7,000 to $61,000 per litre. The 1991–1998 Japanese customs department figures estimate that about 34 metric tonnes of unprocessed agarwood is imported annually, with a cumulative total of 277,396 kilograms. Unprocessed agarwood pieces range from $320 to $22,700 per kilogram, with the highest quality fetching between $9,000 and $272,000 per kilogram. The key port for this trade is Hong Kong, which in English means "Fragrant Harbour," indicating the historical importance of this port as an incense-trading hub.

The essential oil is extracted from the heartwood by hydro, steam, and carbon dioxide distillation. An eighty-year-old tree can produce just 6–9 kilograms of agarwood oil. Steam distillation is the most popular mode of extraction: the wood is converted first into chips, and then cooked in a still to remove the oil. The first distillate is the purest, and most expensive. The oil is kept pure or blended with cheaper essential oils like carnation, sandalwood, geranium, and alcohol.

Aristotle was aware that the wound-healing property of agarwood could be invaluable to soldiers in battle, so he advised his student, Alexander the Great, to conquer lands rich in agarwood trees. Dioscorides mentioned aloes in his encyclopedia of herbs *De Materia Medica* (c. 75 BC).

The resin was believed to have antidepressant, antimicrobial, and aphrodisiac properties. It was also used to treat gout, paralysis, and rheumatism. Its carminative property was used to treat diarrhoea, vomiting, and stomach aches. It is considered to be particularly effective in soothing the nerves and reducing anxiety. Animal research trials have indicated that the plant possesses anticancer and antidepressant properties.

According to Traditional Chinese Medicine, agarwood is rated among the top ten Chinese herbal medicines. It works on three meridians: the kidney, spleen, and stomach. In ancient China, the plant was used to treat digestive problems. It was considered an antioxidant. In combination with *Radix aucklandiae* root, *Lindera strychnifolia* root, immature bitter orange, and other herbs, it was used to promote circulation of qi (life force). Qi flows through twelve meridians on each side of the human body. Meridians can be equated to a three-dimensional network of energy flows connecting various organs and pressure points of the human body.

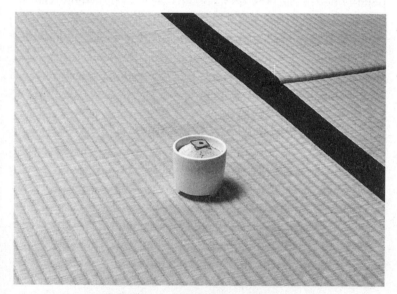

Figure 26 "菖蒲香 (3)" by Gryffindor, own work, licensed under
CC BY-SA 4.0 via Wikimedia Commons

In Tibetan medicine, agarwood is believed to have a calming influence. Black aloeswood is regarded as a minor tranquiliser. When combined with cloves, *Diospyrus kaki* (oriental persimmon) calyx, round cardamom seed, and other drugs, it treats colds, vomiting, and hiccups. The herb can be used in combination with prepared aconite root, cinnamon bark, *Psoraleacorylifolia* fruit, and other herbs, to treat kidney disorders, feeble breath, chronic cough, and asthma. With tangerine peel, *Pinellia ternate* tuber, magnolia bark, *Fructusperillae* fruit, and other drugs, it resolves phlegm, cough, and asthma.

In Ayurvedic medicine, agarwood heartwood is used in popular formulas such as *Chavanprasha, Arimedadi Taila*, and *Mahanarin Taila*. These formulae are used as a cardiac tonic, general tonic, carminative, refrigerant, and to treat sexual disorders. Ayurveda practitioners regard the oil to be beneficial in providing relief in ailments of the chest, head, and skin. There are references to its medicinal use in the *Sushruta Samhita*. In Unani medicine, it is used as a stimulant, laxative, and aphrodisiac. In Japan, the ancient application of agarwood chips for relaxation, meditation, and physical wellness is common in the *Kou-Dou* incense ceremony.

BOSWELLIA (FRANKINCENSE)

One of the most well regarded of the ancient incenses, frankincense has a fresh pine-lemon scent with resinous and woody overtones that emanates from the milky white latex of the stem and branches. The name frankincense comes from the French words *francencens*, which mean "pure incense" or "free lighting." This name originates from the Frank Crusades of the eleventh century, when the Franks were believed to store large quantities of frankincense, for use as incense and medicine. In Arabic, it is called *luban*, which means "white" or "cream" and *olibanum*, which means "oil of Lebanon." In Hebrew, it is called *lebonah*.

Frankincense resin is produced from multiple Boswellia species, the aromas of which vary. The resin is extracted by steam or carbon dioxide distillation. *Boswellia sacra syn B. carterii* has terpenic and pine flavour; *Boswellia papyrifera* is fruity and citrus, with soft orange notes; *Boswellia frereana* has a pungent scent similar to cumin; *Boswellia neglecta* has a soft, earthy, and slightly musty aroma; *Boswellia rivae* is soft, woody, and elegant; and *Boswellia serrata* has fresh lemon, citrus, and pine notes. *B. carterii*, *B. frereana*, *B. papyrifera*, and *B. serrata* of the Burseraceae family are the major sources of frankincense.

B. sacra, with its light lemony scent, is the most prized, and is the species referred to most, in the Bible. This tree grows today in Yemen and Northern Somalia. *Boswellia frereana* and *Boswellia thurifera*, found in Northern Somalia, are sources of the Coptic frankincense that is preferred by the Coptic Church. This too has a pleasant lemony scent, and is also used in Arabian chewing gum.

B. papyrifera is found in Kenya, Ethiopia, Eritrea, and Sudan in Africa. It has an orange scent, and is used to produce the highest quantity of frankincense in the Afro-Arabian region. It is considered as good for the stomach, though it can also cause stomach problems. *B. serrata* grows in the dry regions of India, and yields an orange-scented gum that is lower quality than that of *B. sacra*. The gum is a popular ingredient in Ayurvedic medicine.

China imports the majority of frankincense produced in the world for use in traditional medicine. *B. sacra*-based frankincense was the major import to ancient China, perhaps because of China's proximity to the Silk Route. Decreased production of *B. sacra* trees in Oman and Northern Somalia caused a market share loss of this frankincense.

Multiple references to frankincense in the Bible indicate its importance. The King James Bible contains 113 references to incense and 17 references to frankincense. The Hebrew people blended frankincense with other precious resins like myrrh to make Ketoret, the perfume that was used to prepare the Jewish temple for worship. The three Magi brought gifts of gold, myrrh, frankincense, and spices to Baby Jesus.

As mentioned in Chapter 1, spices were often valued more than gold. Egyptian ladies prepared kohl from burnt frankincense and used that as eyeliner. Tradition has it that Queen Sheba brought frankincense saplings from Arabia for King Solomon. This high premium continued until the nineteenth century AD, when improved logistics, chemical alternatives, and increased supply led to decreased prices.

Frankincense was widely used by people in the Mesopotamian, Arabian, and Mediterranean regions. Itsinebriating, euphoric, and mood-enhancing effects have been recognised for a long time. Some studies have confirmed the psychoactive and antidepressant effects of frankincense incense. The oil aids in treating skin ailments like acne and warts.

The Assyrians associated the incense with the goddess Ishtar and the gods Adonis and Bel (Ratsch, 1998, 92). Frankincense was a natural insecticide used by ancient Egyptians to fumigate wheat and grain stores and deter moths. In Arabia, they burned resin to keep mosquitoes and sand flies away. According to a reference in the Talmud, frankincense was given to intoxicate criminals before putting them to death.

Theophrastus, Dioscorides, and Pliny, all mentioned the medicinal properties of frankincense. Dioscorides, the Roman military physician, used frankincense resin to treat soldiers' wounds. He mentions the resin coming from the incense growing regions of Arabia, which are now in Yemen and Oman, adulterated with gum Arabic and pine resin. Avicenna, the Arabic physician of the eleventh century AD, recommended frankincense to reduce fevers.

In Traditional Chinese Medicine, frankincense (*ru xiang*) has been used for centuries. The first reference to frankincense is in the Chinese medicine book *Mingyi Bielu*, or *Miscellaneous Records of Famous Physicians* (c. 500 AD). It is regarded to have a positive effect on qi. It invigorates the blood, dispels blood stasis, and it treats swelling, wounds, sore muscles, sores and boils, abdominal pain, dysmenorrhea, postpartum abdominal pain, and pain caused by trauma.

Just like other herbal medical formulations, frankincense is used in combination with other herbs. It is used in health care products such as cosmetics, soaps, perfumes, lotions, toothpaste, mouthwashes, and medical ointments. It is also used in varnishes, adhesives, fumigation powders, pastilles, food flavours, chewing gum, and wound plasters. The aroma calms the nerves, enhances spirituality, and aids in meditation, and prayer. However, the WHO has classified frankincense smoke as slightly hazardous.

Boswellia sacra (Omani Luban)

The *B. sacra* (Omani luban) tree is native to Yemen, Oman, and Somalia. It yields the best and most prized frankincense gum. The tree rarely grows taller than 20 feet. It bears whitish yellow flowers. Phytochemical analysis of the essential oil from botanically certified oleogum resin of *B. sacra* show that E-β-cymene and limonene make up 97.3 percent of the oil, followed by sesquiterpene E caryophyllene at 2.7 percent (Al-Harrasi and Al-Saidi, 2008). This analysis further shows a complete absence of diterpenes.

The world's finest *B. sacra* frankincense comes from the Dhofar region in Oman, which lies in the Nejd valley with steep slopes of the rich soil and dense limestone. The climate is dry, hot, and xerophytic. The local Beit Kathir and al Mahra tribes control the frankincense trade, and the best trees are restricted to a small geographic region. Thus, consumers have been forced to look for alternatives. Cheaper substitutes may smell like frankincense, but they do not yield the white smoke that is typical of the pure oleoresin.

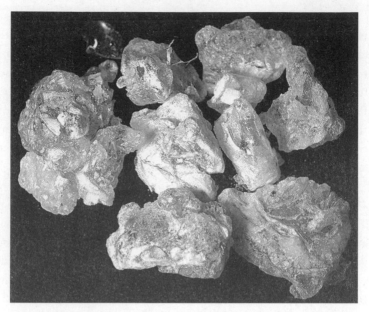

Figure 27 Frankincense from Yemen, "Frankincense 2005-12-31" by snotch,
photo taken by author, licensed under Public Domain via Wikimedia Commons

B. sacra resin exudes from the stem when the bark is either naturally or artificially stripped. Tapping of the resin is done by blazing, or cutting, the tree at multiple points. The resin forms tears, which are left in situ (the place of exudation) to dry, and then collected by gum collectors. The blazes must be refreshed twice annually in spring and fall, to re-open the channel, similar to other resin-yielding trees. The best resin is clear white with a greenish tinge, and it is said to be reserved for the Sultan of Oman. Very little resin is exported.

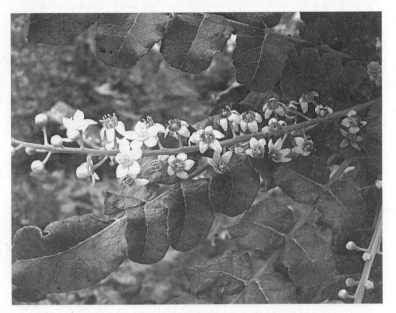

Figure 28 "Boswellia sacra" by Scott Zona from USA,
licensed under CC BY 2.0 via Wikimedia Commons

The entire *B. sacra* frankincense production region is adversely impacted by increasing biotic pressure from increased cattle herds. A lack of forest management and protection has led to exploitation and deforestation of *B. sacra* trees. The International Union for Conservation of Nature has classified the species growing in Oman, Somalia, and Yemen as "near threatened" category, and has declared that the trees in Oman are so heavily harvested, that they no longer flower or produce seed. This has led to rapid depletion of tree stock.

Studies further indicate that the Oman stands suffer from endemism, which diminishes gene pool diversity, and increases the threat of extinction. The absence of a scientific supply chain, inadequate habitat protection, and the geopolitical situation in Yemen and Somalia, has further adversely impacted the habitat.

Medicinal Use of Boswellia Sacra. As previously stated, chewing frankincense gum is common in Arabian countries, especially Saudi Arabia. It is traditionally believed that gum chewing is good for oral hygiene. Studies conducted on five human females aged 25–35 found that chewing frankincense gum for five hours reduced bacterial activity.

The antibacterial, anti-inflammatory, and anticarcinogenic properties of the oleoresin have also been tested and validated in animal trials. Treatment with essential oil of frankincense enhanced cell death and decreased growth of human breast cancer and skin cancer cells, indicating possible pharmaceutical use.

Tests conducted on the fungi *Aspergillus flavus* and *Aspergillus parasiticus* reveal that the resin and oil of *B. sacra* reduces carcinogenic and other deleterious effects of the fungus, validating its traditional use as a food preservative. The essential oil, which is distilled from gum crystals, is used in aromatherapy and massage oils, and sold under various trade formulations. It has a soothing effect on the nerves and takes four to six hours to evaporate, properties which make it a useful fixative in incense making.

Boswellia frereana (Maydi Frankincense)

Maydi Frankincense is found in the northern hilly and limestone-rich regions of Somalia. The trees can grow to a height of eight metres. They have swollen stem bases, a papery flaky outer bark, and a dark inner bark. The reddish green flowers are five millimetres wide and arranged in racemes. Resin is tapped through incisions that penetrate the inner bark. Over time, the exuded white sap crystallises to yellow resin tears on the stems. The tears are then harvested.

Maydi frankincense used to be a major export of Somalia, but the unstable political situation and conflict there hindered its production. Distillation, packing, and branding of resin into essential oil now takes place outside of Somalia, although individual land owners still tap their *B. frereana* trees. Nevertheless, the collection and trade of frankincense is disorganised, just like the business of non-timber forest products in other parts of the world.

Products that generate substantial profits (e.g., tendu leaves in India; saffron in Iran) tend to receive the most attention from governments. Non-timber forest products represent just a fraction of the market, and intermediaries and traders who buy directly from local markets and farmers make most of the profit. About 70–80 percent of gum exports are used in chewing gum manufacturing. The rest is split between China, where it is used mainly for medicinal purposes, and Europe, where it is used as incense in religious ceremonies such as in Coptic Christian churches.

Medicinal uses of Boswellia frereana*. B. frereana* frankincense is relatively low in boswellic acid, compared to *B. sacra, B. payprifera*, and *B. serrata*. Many believe that boswellic acid is responsible for frankincense's many medicinal properties, but modern scientific research does not appear to substantiate this claim. About 70–80 percent of Maydi frankincense is sold to Saudi Arabia for chewing gum. The gum is a crystalline gold colour, and is traditionally regarded to heal ailments of the mouth and stomach, freshen the mouth, and strengthen teeth and gums.

Some believe that the incense enhances brain activity. Scientific studies by Blain et al. (2010) validate the antimicrobial property of *B. frereana*, although it was less than that of *B. sacra*. The anti-inflammatory property of *B. frereana* has also been researched and validated, but further evaluation is needed.

Boswellia papyrifera (African Frankincense)

Boswellia papyrifera grows fairly extensively in Ethiopia, Eritrea, Kenya, and Sudan. This deciduous species is taller than *B. frereana* and *B. sacra*, reaching 12 metres, with a clear bole. The species grows on steep escarpments in locations where other species find it difficult to survive. It thus helps protect hill sides by providing much needed soil cover and could perhaps be used in soil stabilisation.

The soft timber is suitable for plywood and matchwood and is used locally as small timber. The plant bears sweetly scented white to pink flowers and red capsular fruit. The bark is whitish to pale brown and flaking, similar to *B. sacra* and *B. frereana*. Like other Boswellia species that produce frankincense, the resin channels are located just below the inner bark. The tapping blaze is a square of 2.5 centimetres that is made only on the surface at a depth of 1 millimetre. The tree can be tapped 8–12 times during dry periods, and trees can yield resin for 50–60 years.

African Frankincense from Ethiopia is classified into five grades based on granule size, colour, and purity. The first grade includes white granules that are 6 mm or larger in diameter; the second includes 4–6 mm granules; the third includes 2–4 mm granules; the fourth includes brown and black granules of any size; and the fifth grade is powder mixed with bark.

B. papyrifera frankincense has a fruity and citrus aroma with a predominantly soft orange flavour. *B. papyrifera* comprises 90 percent of exported frankincense; *B. neglecta* and *B. rivae* comprise the rest. Most frankincense produced from the region is exported to China for use in traditional medicine. The distilled oil is exported to Europe for use in incense in Orthodox and Roman Catholic ceremonies, though sandalwood is a popular alternative.

B. papyrifera forms the bulk of the world supply of frankincense today, though over exploitation of the resin has led to its rapid depletion. Setting of seed and regeneration, which is already difficult given the preference of the species to inhabit steep escarpments, is further jeopardised by overgrazing and trampling by goats, sheep, and other fauna, and this hardens the forest floor.

Additionally, inadequately trained harvesters damage the already threatened trees, indicating a lack of sound silvicultural practices for *B. papyrifera.*

Studies by Rijkers et al. (2006) have revealed that tapping for frankincense leads to reduction in seeding, and regeneration of *B. papyrifera.* Reduced saplings and seedlings on the forest floor are an early sign of degradation and decline of a crop. Although Tadesse et al. (2007) estimate that 1.5 million hectares of *B. papyrifera* remains available, it has been estimated that more than 170,000 hectares of *B. papyrifera* have been destroyed by fire over the last 20 years. Forest fires, either caused by humans or weather, are one reason for this decline. Fires occur in dry months when tapping is in full swing. The resin is inflammable. Ground fires tend to rapidly escalate into crown fires, which are more destructive to the ecology, and cause rapid depletion of the site.

In Eritrea, frankincense exports have dropped to just 25 percent of their levels in the 1970s. War, a lack of governance, and poor forest and habitat management have further aggravated the situation. Thus, TRAFFIC has put *B. papyrifera* in the endangered species category.

Medicinal uses of Boswellia papyrifera. A comparative phytochemical analysis of *B. papyrifera, B. neglecta,* and *B. rivae* has revealed that *B. papyrifera* contains diterpenes and nortriterpenes, and the other two are composed of triterpenes. Studies on rats exposed to *B. papyrifera* and *B. carterii* smoke indicate that prolonged exposure to frankincense smoke has a negative impact on the human reproductive system. *B. papyrifera* and *B. carterii* resins are effective against a range of pathogenic bacteria.

Sediqui et al. (2014) conducted a clinical trial on 80 multiple sclerosis patients in an Iranian hospital and found that the resin had a positive effect on the visual-cognitive faculties, although no impact on verbal cognition was noticed. Experiments on rats also indicate that the plant improved learning abilities of rats. These findings validate the traditional uses of frankincense for treating mental disorders.

Boswellia Serrata (Indian Frankincense, *Salai*)

Boswellia serrata is a mid-sized tree found in the drier regions of Northern and Central India. Locally, the tree is also called *salai*. The trees can reach a height of 15 metres and width of 1.5 metres. The bole of the tree is three to five metres, rendering it unsuitable for use as timber. The tree rarely grows in pure stands, and is often mixed with other dry deciduous tree species, like *Anogeissus latifolia*, *Acacia leucophloea*, and Terminalia species. The trees are found on steeper slopes of relatively thin soil, and on flat terrain.

B. serrata is one of the four major frankincense-yielding trees from these regions. The resin was extensively traded and used by ancient societies of Rome, Greece, China, India, Arabia, and the Americas, and it is still used in cultural and religious events in these regions. Aromatic resin exudes from gaps in the bark of this species. *B. serrata* is used in India more as a medicinal plant than for incense. It is extensively used in Ayurveda.

B. serrata extract is collected by tapping from mixed forests. It is exported to Europe and North America, and used in aromatherapy, massage, natural perfumes, creams, and incense. Its medicinal and essential oil uses are not sufficient for the species to be a preferred agroforestry species, such as pine. Thus, nearly all sap collection is from wild-growing trees. The tapping method is similar to other Boswellia species. It entails making a shallow incision in the bark, and collecting the exudate. No tapping is done in the monsoon season. According to forest regulations in India, only trees larger than 90 centimetres in diameter at breast height are permitted to be tapped.

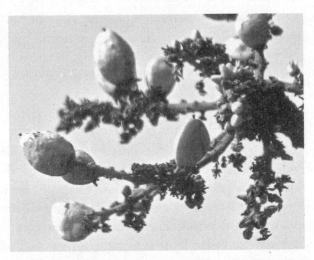

Figure 29 "Boswellia serrata (Salai) in Kinnarsani WS, AP W2 IMG 5840" by J.M. Garg, own work, licensed under GFDL via Wikimedia Commons

Medicinal Uses of Boswellia serrata. The species has an anti-inflammatory action used to treat liver inflammation, stomach ulcers, rheumatoid arthritis, osteoarthritis, bronchial asthma, and Crohn's disease. It is said to be particularly effective in treating painful knee inflammations. Traditionally, healers use the species extensively to treat a variety of arthritis and inflammatory conditions.

Trials and research indicate that the plant could emerge as an alternative to non-steroidal anti-inflammatory drugs, which are associated with a high prevalence of gastrointestinal and cardiovascular adverse effects in humans. In 2002, the European Medicines Agency classified *B. serrata*-based medicine as an "orphan drug" that could be used to treat peritumoural brain edema.

Animal trials have been indicated anticonvulsant properties that could be useful in treating epilepsy. The species may help treat a range of cancer-causing tumours, including brain tumours.

The active ingredients isolated from the species include Boswellic acids, monoterpenes, diterpenes, triterpenes, tetracyclic triterpenic acids, and pentacyclic triterpenes. The oleo-gum resins contain 30–60 percent resins, 5–10 percent essential oils, and the rest is polysaccharides.

STACTE (*NATAF*)

Stacte, known in Hebrew as *nataf*, is one of the four ingredients in Holy Incense referred to in Exodus 35:34. As with most Biblical and other religious references to herbs and plants, the botany of the plant from which the spice, incense, or medicine was extracted, has been a matter of considerable debate and discussion. In this case, some say that stacte is another name for myrrh. Both are gum exudates, collected in the form of tears. Scholars have referenced Herodotus and Pliny to support this claim. The plant apparently grew in the Mediterranean. Pliny mentions it in his Book XII of *Natural Historia*. In Book LV of *Natural Historia*, he states, "The Syrians value this gum highly, and use it medicinally as a demulcent in pectoral complaints, and also in perfumery." Perhaps this fragrant gum was collected in the same manner as myrrh, or perhaps it was another tree gum called tragacanth.

In view of the lack of archaeological evidence as to the source of stacte, we must rely on circumstantial evidence. Pliny mentions that stacte was found in the region that is now Syria. Herodotus notes that different kinds of "storax" were actively traded during his time. Storax was an aromatic spice used as incense and in medicine.

An Egyptian perfume formula from 1200 BC consisted of "Storax, Labdanum, Galbanum, Frankincense, Myrrh, Cinnamon, Cassia, Honey, Raisins" (Keville and Green, 2008) Rosenmeuller (1840) records that "the Greeks also called stacte, a species of Storax gum, which Dioscorides described as transparent like a tear, and resembling myrrh."

From at least 500 BC to 1000 AD, an active trade in spices existed between the Arabia Peninsula, India, Malaku (modern day Indonesia), Northern Africa, Greece, Rome, and Israel. It is probable that stacte, referred to as one of the ingredients in the Holy Incense mentioned in Exodus 30:34, could be storax. However, it is highly unlikely that it is synonymous with myrrh, as there are extensive references to myrrh throughout the Old and the New Testaments, and it is thus unlikely that myrrh and stacte would be used interchangeably.

Another contender for stacte are species belonging to the genus Styrax. *Styrax benzoin*, *Styrax benzoides*, and *Styrax tonkinensis* are three species found extensively in Malacca, in modern Indonesia. They all are sources of pleasant-smelling gum. *S. benzoin* gum is used as incense in churches and mosques today. The popular name for this oleoresin is gum Benjamin. According to Wikipedia, the name *benzoin* probably derives from the Arabic *luban jawai* (Javan frankincense). Styrax is still used in the Middle East as an air freshener. Maybe, as Dioscorides said, multiple types of storax or styrax were traded in the region. It is therefore likely that the stacte-like frankincense came from multiple plants.

STYRAX OFFICINALIS

Styrax inhabits eastern Mediterranean countries across Italy, Turkey, and Israel. A styrax variety also grows in California in the United States. In Israel, styrax grows in the Judean and Samarian mountains on Mount Carmel, and in Herman, the Upper Jordan, and other northern valleys. Styrax often has a shrub-like appearance but is classified as a tree and can grow to five metres in height. It inhabits dry rocky slopes in woods, thickets, and near streams. This deciduous tree has white flowers that emanate a citrus fragrance, attracting many bees and insects. The smoke from the tree is aromatic, but toxic.

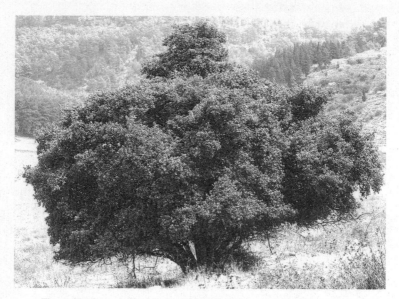

Figure 30 "Styrax officinalis tree" by Eitan F., own work, licensed under
CC BY-SA 3.0 via Wikimedia Commons

The Israeli species does not yield resin. Some claim that the absence of resin in the Israeli varieties is a consequence of genetic changes, but there is no evidence to support this theory. Seven of the eight ancient Greek Hymns of Orpheus mention storax 13 times, which is only slightly fewer than the most popular aromatic spice, frankincense. Storax was likely a highly valued aromatic resin. An essential oil produced from *S. officinalis* seed in Turkey is used in some Roman Catholic churches in Europe.

A branch from the tree is said to have been used as a staff by Moses. Styrax and benzoin balsams have been used since ancient times by Romans and others (Gianno et al., 1990; Modugno et al., 2006) to treat chronic infections of the respiratory tract. The plant has therapeutic and pharmacological properties as a disinfectant and expectorant.

Avicenna's *Law of Medicine* indicates that styrax resin mixed with antibiotic substances and hardening materials is a good dental restorative material. Nowadays, the resin is used as a fixative in perfumes and as a filler and flavour-enhancer in cosmetics and foods (Fernandez et al., 2003, 2006; Castel et al., 2006).

STYRAX BENZOIN (SUMATRA BENZOIN)

Styrax benzoin inhabits the Sumatran region of Indonesia, India, Myanmar, Thailand, Laos, and Malaysia. It is grown as an ornamental shade tree in West Africa. It grows to a height of 12 metres. The tree is a source of benzoin resin. Sumatra benzoin is produced from styrax benzoin on the Sumatra islands of Indonesia. The resin is set in blocks of a dull reddish or grayish-brown colour. The balsamic resin has a strong storax-like odour, quite distinct from the vanilla odour of the Siamese variety.

The Siamese variety of benzoin is produced from *Styrax tonkinensis*, a species in Vietnam, Thailand and Laos, and Cambodia. *S. tonkinensis* is vanilla scented, with a reddish yellow outside and milky white inside. It grows to more than 20 metres in height. Much of the benzoin produced from these trees has impurities and is used primarily in manufacturing. The higher-quality benzoin is used in perfumes.

The FAO (2001) estimates that 50 metric tonnes of Siam's benzoin are exported annually from Laos and Vietnam. Pure benzoin exports are half that amount. China produces some benzoin, but it is largely consumed locally and not exported. Both Siamese and Sumatra benzoins are popular in incense and perfume. It blends well with frankincense, sandalwood, cedar, and citrus oils.

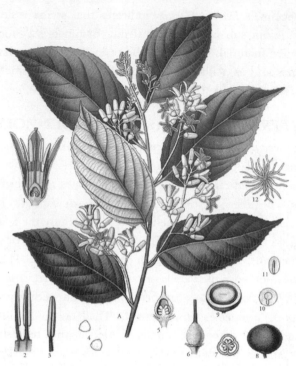

Figure 31 *Styrax benzoin* by Franz Eugen Köhler

Extraction of resin is done by making a deep incision with an axe on the trunk of the tree, when it reaches seven years of age. The wound must be deep enough to expose the cambium canals. The sap is then dried for about four weeks, and the tears are collected and packed in tins or boxes. The first three years of tapping yield the best resin, though the tree continues to yield benzoin for another 10–12 years. At the end of the tree's life, it is cut down and its resin scraped off.

The average annual resin yield from a tree in Sumatra is 1.5 kilograms. A 2001 Food and Agriculture Organisation (FAO) study of Indonesian export data estimates the annual export of Sumatra benzoin at 1,000 metric tonnes. Most *S. benzoin* resin is used by the cosmetic and food industries. Benzoic acid is used as a food flavouring and preservative. In Indonesia, the product is sold as frankincense, although true frankincense comes from Boswellia species. This nomenclature only adds to the confusion regarding the actual origin of stacte.

Papyrus records from ancient Egypt indicate that benzoin resin was mixed with other aromatic resins like pine, juniper, cypress, galbanum, and labdanum, to create an aromatic powder that Egyptian dancers applied to their heads. Benzoin is used as a fragrance by Indonesian Muslims also. In the Middle East, an incense of scented wood chips called *Bakhoor* contains benzoin. *Bakhoor* is used on coal fires to produce a powerful aroma, and is part of the ancient Arabic tribal tradition of living in the outdoors. Benzoin is also used as incense in Orthodox Christian and Greek Christian churches.

Traditionally, *S. benzoin* resin is diluted or blended with other resins, and herbs. In aromatherapy, benzoin has a calming influence on the body, but it can cause contact dermatitis. It is a mild stimulant and antiseptic, and it is used to treat skin irritations such as itchiness, dryness, and redness after blending it with oil.

The oil is blended in cream, and is useful in cuts, wounds, and acne. It is helpful in treating psoriasis and has carminative properties. When taken internally, it is a rapidly absorbed mild expectorant, diuretic, and urinary antiseptic. Benzoin is also used in steam treatments for laryngitis, bronchitis, and asthma. It is sold as a throat and lung decongestant called "Friar's balsam." People take benzoin by mouth to relieve swollen gums and herpes sores.

Benzoin is used in combination with other herbs like aloe, storax, and tolu balsam to relieve aches and arthritis pain. Benzoin has well established uses in both allopathic, and traditional forms of medicine.

There are references to Sumatra and Siam benzoins in allopathic and traditional forms of medicines. British, Chinese,

French, Italian, Japanese, and American pharmacopoeias refer the use of an inhalant with steam for relief of cough, laryngitis, bronchitis, and upper respiratory diseases.

The British pharmacopoeia (1993) specifies use of Sumatra benzoin in inhalation and compound tinctures. The American pharmacopoeia (1994) also describes a compound benzoin tincture, although it does not specify the type of benzoin. The Body Shop chain sells a skin lotion containing lavender oil, sandalwood, vetivert, patchouli, and benzoin. The Chinese pharmacopoeia (1992) mentions benzoin preparations of pills and powders to restore consciousness, activate blood flow, and relieve pain.

Benzoin contains benzoic acid and cinnaminic acid. Benzoic acid is a food preservative, flavouring agent, and flavour booster that increases the spiciness of other flavours, especially vanilla or cassia. In syrups, it enhances turbidity. Sumatran benzoin has substantial amounts of cinnamates, which is a component of cocoa and other chocolate-flavoured products. It is especially popular in Denmark and Sweden, where it is used to glaze confections such as chocolate eggs. In Japan, where it is approved for use, benzoin is employed as a chewing gum base. It is recognised as a food and tobacco flavouring agent in the United States.

GALBANUM (FERULA GALBANIFLUA)

Ferula galbaniflua syn F gummosa is found in Iran, Southern Russia, Afghanistan, and Turkey. It is a perennial that grows to a height of one metre. The plant bears umbelliferus yellow flowers arranged in a panicle. The gum resin is extracted by wounding the root or lower part of the stem. The resin that oozes out of the wound is collected around two weeks after wounding, by which time the exudates have hardened into a crystalline substance. The chemical constituents of galbanum are monoterpenes (α and β pinene), sabinene, limonene, undecatriene, and pyrazines.

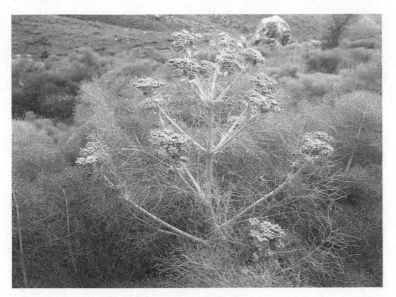

Figure 32 "Goli Lo" by Pirehelokan, own work

Galbanum is one of the four essential ingredients of the Holy Incense mentioned in Exodus 30:34 and Ecclesiastes 24:14–15. It was one of the ingredients of Ketoret, the Jewish Holy Incense that was burned in the Tabernacle in the first and second Jewish Temple at Jerusalem.

The current widely accepted source of galbanum is *Ferula gummosa*, which is synonymous with *Ferula galbaniflua*, though other species also yield galbanum. It has an acute and unpleasant smell, hence its nickname "devils dung" in English, which makes one, wonder about its selection for use in ancient incense. Galbanum was likely a fixative in ancient perfumes, and it is still used as such today. Fixatives do not need to be sweet smelling. Fixatives instead enhance, and prolong the scent of perfumes. The plant that produces galbanum has chemical compounds similar to the pungent *asafoetida*, a spice that is popular in Indian cuisine.

Nomads of South-western Iran have traditionally used the plant as an antidiarrheal. Ancient Iranian medical literature refers to it as an anticonvulsant, antispasmodic, expectorant, and wound treatment. These treatments have been studied in trials on rats, but they have not been validated in clinical trials.

The resin's antibacterial action was studied, but little activity was detected. Scientists have also studied the spasmolytic action of the essential oil against part of the intestine. In Iranian traditional medicine, an oleo-gum-resin obtained from *F.gummosa* is popular for treating various disorders that include stomachache, cholera, diarrhoea, epilepsy, inflammation, and pain. In a review of the species conducted by Nabavi et al. (2012) in Iran, the anti-oxidant action of the gum was studied, and validated.

Galbanum was actively traded in pre- and post-Biblical times. It was sourced largely from Mesopotamia and Turkey. Today, these countries continue to be major producers. Galbanum is not known to grow in Israel, and the Israeli plants database does not mention it. This supports the theory that galbanum, like many spices referred in the Old and the New Testaments, were imported into the region. Galbanum was exported from the galbanum production regions of Mesopotamia, Asia Minor, India, China, Israel, the Mediterranean, and Egypt.

Galbanum resin comes from the root and lower part of the stem of Ferula species that grow in Iran, Afghanistan, Turkey, and neighboring areas. Three species, *F. gummosa*, *Ferula rubricaulis*, and *F. ceratophylla*, are known to yield galbanum resin. The first two grow in Iran, and *F. ceratophylla* is native to Turkestan.

Resin is harvested from trees in the wild. The collected gum is sold in village markets, where traders sell it to wholesalers who, in turn, export it to processing units, mostly in Europe and the United States. Iran is the largest producer of gum resin, at about 15 metric tonnes (FAO 2006). Turkey also produces substantial quantities of galbanum, but accurate estimates are difficult to obtain, as most data are aggregates of multiple commodities.

There are two varieties of resin. Persian galbanum is soft. Its yellowish tears are honey-like, viscous, translucent, and yellow to red in colour. It is used in incense and fragrance making. Levant galbanum is hard. The exudate lumps can be broken easily. The crude gum contains "foots," which is the trade name for gum with impurities of sand, water, insects, and wood chips.

The product is purified by straining during the summer. Steam distillation yields 15–25 percent oil. A 40–50 percent extract can be obtained by solvent extraction that produces a resinoid. Pourable grades of the resinoid are obtained by extracting the crude gum with a perfume diluent, such as diethyl phthalate or benzyl benzoate. The yields vary, depending on the quantity of "foots" in the gum. Levant galbanum is mostly used in pharmaceuticals and industrials.

Although galbanum resin and oil are used to flavour food including baked goods, candy, and ice creams, its main use is in perfume. Perfumers use galbanum as a strong top note in "green" fragrances, and as a base note in combination with musk and chypre elements, such as oakmoss and pine.

On its own, galbanum has a brash and rough character, but it provides a traditional green note to florals like hyacinth, gardenia, narcissus, iris, and violet. The following fragrances contain galbanum: Chanel No. 19, Guerlain Vol De Nuit, Cartier Must, Balmain Vent Vert, Fresh Galbanum Patchouli, Prince Matchabelli Cachet, Il Profumo Chocolat, Bill Blass Nude, Les Parfums de Rosine Rose d'Amour, Molinard Les Fleurs, Fleur de Figuier, Issey Miyake A Scent, Prada Infusion d'Iris, Chloe Eau de Fleurs Capucine, and Azzaro Couture. For men's fragrances, galbanum is included in Etienne Aigner Private Number, Serge Lutens Borneo 1834, Aramis Devin, Miller Harris Patchouli, Laura Biagiotti Roma Per Uomo, and Versace Blue Jeans for Men (https://en.wikipedia.org/wiki/Galbanum).

Galbanum is mentioned in the medicinal works of Hippocrates and Pliny the Elder. Galbanum was one of at least 36 ingredients used by Mithridates (c. 132–163 BC) as medicine. Mithridates VI was a Roman who ruled over Pontus, now in the Anatolian region of Turkey. His father, Mithridates V, was said to have been poisoned, and killed. Mithridates VI administered herb-based poisons to himself in small quantities to render himself immune from poisoning. This antidote, which contained galbanum, became known as *Antidotum Mithridaticum*, or Theriac.

Dioscorides prescribed the milky juice of galbanum for ulcers, coughs, convulsions, ruptures, headaches, stomach pains, menstrual cramps, toothaches, snakebites, and labour pain. Rubbed on the eyes as an ointment, it improved eyesight. Taken with honey, galbanum was regarded as a remedy for indigestion and flatulence.

The Assyrians used it as a fumigant. Galbanum essential oil, usually blended with other oils, was used to treat wounds, scars, inflammations, and skin disorders. Athletes used it to relieve pulled and sore muscles, cramps, and aching feet. It also relaxes the nerves and muscles while ridding the body of toxic substances. In a tincture with alcohol, it is effective in getting rid of head lice.

In modern aromatherapy, the essential oil of galbanum is used in bath and massage oils. It is believed to impact the body, mind, and spirit. It relieves muscular ache and swollen lymph glands. The oil has analgesic properties and helps to treat cuts, wounds, abscesses, and wrinkles. It is useful in providing relief for cough, bronchitis, asthma, and lung infections.

NARDOSTACHYS JATAMANSI (SPIKENARD)

Nardostachys jatamansi is a flowering herb found in the Himalayan region at altitudes of 3000–5000 metres. The plant grows to a height of one metre and has bell-shaped pink flowers. The rhizomes are crushed and distilled to yield a long-lasting amber-coloured aromatic oil used in incense, perfume, and herbal medicine. The essential oil has a green, moderately powerful, medicinal, and herbaceous top note that is spicy and sweet. The middle notes are of clove and ginger, with rich earth, wet wood, and dried leaf undertones.

Spikenard essential oil blends well with pine, lavender, patchouli, and vetiver oil. The oil is non-toxic and non-irritating on the skin. It is often used in combination with other short-lived scents like rose. Roots and rhizomes contain a variety of sesquiterpenes and coumarins.

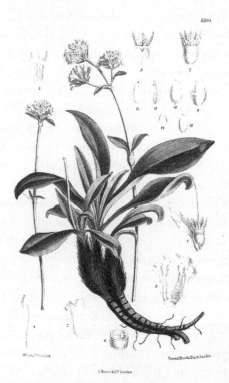

Figure 33 "Nardostachys grandiflora" by Joseph Dalton Hooker (1817–1911)

The collection and harvesting of *N. jatamansi* is done before the first snow, usually from May to July. Harvesting too early can cause a year's growth loss, because the plant's growing period starts after the spring snowmelt, and continues until November. The rhizomes are physically uprooted, which decreases their numbers, and availability. Thus, *N. jatamansi* was added to the Convention on International Trade in Endangered Species of Wild Fauna and Flora list in 1997 at the request of India, followed by further restrictions in 2007.

Manufactured preparations, such as powders, pills, extracts, and teas are still permitted to be traded, but bulk herb materials (whole and sliced roots) are restricted. Given the fragile ecology of the Himalayan region, any relaxation of these restrictions could lead to rapid depletion of the species. Yet, Nepal continues to export substantial quantities of *N. jatamansi* rhizomes to India. Olsen (2005) estimates that 100–500 metric tonnes of air-dried rhizomes are exported annually from Nepal to India.

Tibet exports 50–100 metric tonnes of rhizomes to Nepal. Mulliken and Crofton (2008) evaluated Nepalese Customs and Exports data and estimate that in 2000–2001, 21 metric tonnes of essential oil were exported from Nepal. However, with the high-quality alternatives (e.g., *Selinum vaginatum, Valeriana wallichi*) available today, demand for spikenard essential oil in Jewish and Christian ceremonies has decreased, though it is still blended with other essential oils like frankincense and rose.

Efforts to artificially propagate the species have shown mixed results, because it is not economically attractive for collectors to switch from wild to commercial cultivation. Some estimates indicate that the collector's share in the final price of the product is lower than two percent.

These efforts are driven by the Indian Medicinal Plant Board, which encourages nursery development and plantation, through grants and education. However, the Board has not managed the supply chain effectively or established financially rewarding business models, mainly because of its bureaucratic and institutional deficiencies. This experience with spikenard conservation and propagation has exposed larger concerns about the Board's ability to manage herbal product cultivation and management. Coordination between cultivators and industry is minimal, and the trade has not changed in millennia.

Religious literature indicates that spikenard is from the root of *N. jatamansi*, which was a valuable spice in ancient Egypt. The oil of spikenard was used to anoint priests and kings, and in the Egyptian incense Kyphi. Archaeologists have discovered terracotta vessels containing spikenard, sealed with cloth and beeswax, in Pakistan and India. It was imported to the Mediterranean from India, via the spice and silk routes.

In Greece and Rome, spikenard was used to make a popular unguent called nardinium, which helped to meditate and calm the nerves. When mixed with olive oil, it was used for consecration, dedication, and worship, a practice that continues even now. It was also an ingredient in the Jewish Ketoret incense. As previously mentioned, incense was burned in Jewish temples to mask the smell from animal sacrifices. Traditionally, spikenard and other incenses were also used to anoint visitors' forehead and feet, which were often covered in dirt from traveling.

The Bible as well as the Old Testament mentions Spikenard, or nard, at least seven times. Song of Solomon 1:10–13 alludes to the romance associated with this incense. It is said that the cost of a pound of spikenard was 300 to 400 denari. The daily wage of labour at that time was one denari. Thus, a pound of spikenard cost more than a year's wages. Israel's King Hezekaih kept "the spices, and the precious ointment" (2 Kings 20:13) together with silver and gold in the royal treasure chamber. The high price is reiterated in John 12:3.

N. jatamansi is said to be useful for disorders of the digestive and respiratory systems and is a sedative. In aromatherapy, spikenard is used to treat inflammation, insomnia, migraine, stress, and allergies. The root is used to treat insomnia, blood and circulatory system problems, and mental disorders.

In Ayurveda, spikenard is mentioned in all major herbal medicine treatises of Sushruta, Charaka, and others, as a herb that calms nerves, reduces blood pressure, and treats nervous system ailments such as epilepsy. According to the High Altitude Plant Physiology Research Centre, the rhizome is used in about 26 Ayurvedic medicines. An Ayurvedic medicine called Ayush 56 is manufactured in India to treat hysteria, convulsions, and epilepsy. This Ayurvedic formulation has a number of ingredients that include *N. jatamansi* extracts.

According to Traditional Chinese Medicine, *N. jatamansi* is effective in treating pain relief and turgid chest, and in regulating qi (Zhang et al., 1994). Xiang Pu mentions that spikenard incense has a calming effect on the body, and mentions a combination of sandalwood, spikenard, and aloeswood. In Bhutan, spikenard is primarily used as incense during religious rites. Japanese temples use spikenard to produce incense sticks.

In Unani, the species is regarded as a cardiotonic, hepatotonic, analgesic, and diuretic. Many of the resins used in Biblical and Greek periods that include spikenard had antiseptic properties with long-lasting effects, particularly useful to treat and mask the odour from patients with sepsis and putrefied wounds.

There are references to spikenard in the works of Dioscorides, Theophrastus, and Pliny. Dioscorides called it *Gangitis*, derived from the River Ganga that flows down the Himalayas across the Northern Indo-Gangetic plains, into the Bay of Bengal. Arabic and Persian physicians refer to *N. jatamansi* as *Sumbul-i-Hindi* (Indian spike). They distinguish the species from another spikenard-yielding species in Turkey and Egypt that they called *Sumbul-i-Rumi* or *Ikliti*, which has been identified as *Valeriana celtica*. Although it is a substitute for *N. jatamansi*, there is a difference in aroma between the two species. *N. jatamansi* has a pleasant musk-like aroma, and is used in fragrances, such as women's hair and bath products, and it is a major ingredient in incense, and Indian massage oils. *V. celtica*, on the other hand, is foul smelling like dirty socks.

The medicinal properties of spikenard have been widely studied, and several experimental results have validated its traditional medicinal use. Many trials have indicated that the plant has a positive impact on the central nervous system, liver, and cardiac systems, and the plant shows positive results as an anticonvulsant, hyperlipidemic, and cardiotonic agent (Salim et al., 2003; Rucker et al., 1979; Prabhu et al., 1994; Mishra et al., 1995; Metkar et al., 1999, Lyle et al., 2009). Hair growth in rats increased when treated with *N. jatamansi*. Experiments on rats indicate that *N. jatamansi* has neuroprotective properties and may be useful in treating neurological ailments like amnesia, though there are no human clinical trials to support this. It also is said to possess nootropic properties that improve memory, mood, and behaviour.

CROCUS SATIVA (SAFFRON)

Crocus sativus (saffron) is a small flowering herb that is 15 to 30 centimetres tall and distributed across central Asia, Iran, Mediterranean, Europe, Asia (largely Kashmir and Afghanistan), Northern Africa, and North America, in areas with hot dry summers and cold winters.

This perennial herb is unknown in the wild, and has been cultivated for more than 3,000 years. It is believed to be a mutant of the wild *C. cartwrightianus* of the Iridaceae family. *C. sativus* is a triploid and the plant grows 20–30 centimetres tall. Its key constituents are safranal, crocin, cartenoids, glycoside forms, terpene derivatives, anthocyanins, flavonoids, the vitamins riboflavin and thiamine, amino acids, proteins, and starch.

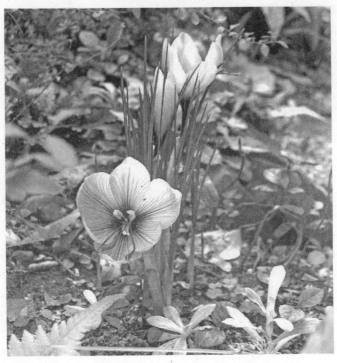

Figure 34 "Crocus sativus1" by KENPEI

The flowers do not produce fertile seeds, so propagation is done with corms, or bulbs, which lie beneath the surface. These corms, which are poisonous to animals, average approximately 0.1 metre in size. Large corms tend to yield more flowers, and thus more saffron. Shoots and blue flowers emanate from the centre of the corm. A single corm can yield saffron for 4–12 years.

The plant does not require much water. In the Khorasan area of Iran, the plantations are irrigated, whereas Kashmiri plantations are mostly rain fed. The cultivation area is ploughed and weeded regularly, until the picking cycle, which lasts four days. Flowers are picked by hand, and then, the plants wither in summer as bulbs go dormant. The aromatic saffron spice is produced by removing the stamens and styles, and placing them on a mesh over a coal or wood fire to dry. A hectare of saffron flowers can yield up to 25 kilograms of saffron, but it takes approximately 150,000 flowers to produce 1 kilogram of saffron. The FAO estimates that saffron requires 200 person-days per hectare for collection, and management. Saffron generally does not store well for longer twelve months. In areas with high labour costs, like Spain, France, Italy, the United Kingdom, and Switzerland, its production is not cost-effective.

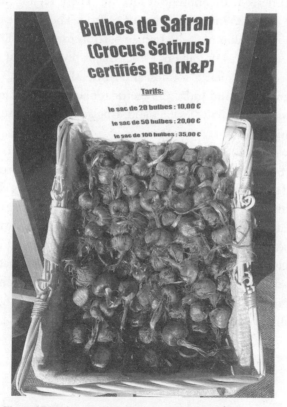

Figure 35 "Safran - Saffron bulbs" by RudolfSimon, own work

According to FAO statistics, Iran is the largest producer and exporter of saffron, with 79,394 hectares in the Khorasan, Fars, and Kerman provinces devoted to saffron cultivation. This is in part because U.S. oil sanctions against Iran have resulted in shifting focus from oil to non-oil exports like saffron. The industry is popular among local communities. The Iranian economic model emphasises sharing profits with growers and collectors, who receive 65 percent of the end-consumer price as a wage.

In the Iranian saffron-producing areas, saffron accounts for up to 70 percent of household income. These regions annually produce about 239 metric tonnes of saffron. The FAO estimates that the total value of 2012 Iranian saffron exports (130 metric tonnes) was US $419 million. Other major producers of saffron are Greece (5.7 metric tonnes annually), Morocco (2.3 metric tonnes annually), and India (2.3 metric tonnes annually), followed by Turkmenistan, Italy, Switzerland, England, France, the United States, and Spain.

Iran exports 84 percent of its saffron, nearly half of which goes to Spain, which is currently the world's major reprocessing and packaging centre for saffron. Reprocessing includes cleaning, sorting, drying, and packaging. Spain's saffron-processing capacity is estimated by FAO to be 220 metric tonnes per annum. Spain, Italy, and the United States are the largest importers of saffron. Saffron is an expensive spice, thus adulteration with petals and flower, such as safflower and marigold, is common. It is cultivated for its fragrance, dye, and culinary uses. It is used in Italian, Greek, and Arabic confections, desserts, and curries.

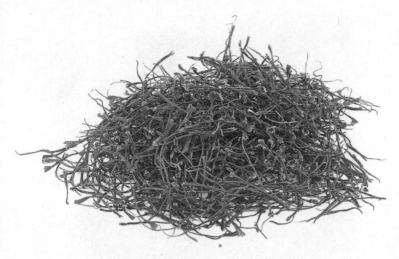

Figure 36 "Safran-Weinviertel Niederreiter 2
Gramm 8285" by Hubertl, own work

Saffron is perhaps the most expensive and ancient among incenses known to man. Saffron-based pigments were probably used to make stencil prints on the walls of caves by earliest of cave inhabitants around 30000 BC. But the earliest saffron dye pigments used in paintings probably goes back to the Minoan period. In Crete in 1450 BC, a volcanic eruption buried the Minoan palaces and buildings in a cloud of dust, where they remained until their discovery by archaeologists. A building called Xestes 3 in Akrotiri, Greece has several frescoes of girls and women gathering saffron flowers, and bringing them to a goddess seated on a three-tiered platform on a cushion of saffron. Another fresco from the same site shows a woman's bleeding foot being treated with saffron. These frescoes indicate that saffron was perhaps collected locally from the wild. The species shown was probably *Crocus cartwrightianus.*

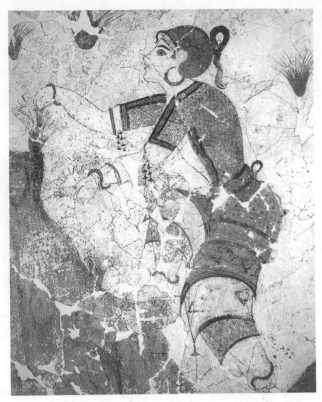

Figure 37 Saffron Gatherers, "Cueilleuse de safran, fresque, Akrotiri, Grèce" by unknown, from Le Musée absolu, Phaidon, 10-2012

Saffron was imported into ancient Egypt and surrounding areas from Crete, and its primary uses were as a dye, and perfume. Barber (1994) observes in *Women's Work: the First 20,000 Years,* that saffron was used to dye women's garments from 3000 BC to 1100 BC, producing a yellow colour ranging from radiant warm yellow, to deep orange-red. Saffron and other aromatic spices were often scattered on pillows and sheets for their aroma and freshness. The spice was mixed with olive oil to scent clothes and hair.

Until the reign of Ramses III, the final layer of the mummification process included a saffron-dyed shroud. It is believed that Cleopatra infused her baths with saffron before sexual encounters. The Ebers papyrus mentions saffron as a plant of medicinal value. It recommends saffron powder blended with beer as a poultice for women in difficult labour and recognises saffron as a diuretic.

There are references to saffron in the tablets and scrolls from the Library of Nineveh during the reign Assyrian king Ashurbanipal (668–627 BC). These tablets are now preserved in the British Museum in London. The spice was collected from flowers found in the wild. Experts believe that *C. cartwrightianus* is the precursor to the cultivated saffron variety *Crocus sativa*, which emerged as a mutation around 1700 BC.

Saffron was also one of the most valued and most expensive aromatic spices of Greco-Roman times. The Greeks called it the "Blood of Hercules." It was used as ritual incense, and regarded as a protective amulet. It was associated with fertility and romance, and nobles used it to perfume clothes, and baths. Homer states that Greek gods Zeus and Jupiter lay on a bed of saffron to enhance amorous emotions. Dioscorides, the Greek physician, mentions the aphrodisiac properties of saffron. It is also mentioned as a ritual incense in the Orphic mysteries of the cult of Dionysus.

Alexander the Great became enamored of saffron in the fourth century BC during his campaign for the conquest of Persia. He used the spice in his baths, perhaps after he defeated Cyrus the Great, and brought the saffron-producing regions of Persia under his control. He believed that saffron helped heal wounds and was good for the skin. Active trade via the Spice and Silk Routes led to increased popularity of saffron.

Shen Nung, a ruler in China (c. twenty-seventh or twenty-eighth century BC) and regarded as the father of Chinese medicine, described medicinal uses of more than 300 herbs, including saffron, in one of the earliest of the extant Materia Medica called the *Divine Husbandsman's Materia Medica*, compiled in the first century AD. There is also reference to saffron in Chinese herbalist Wan Zhen's (c. third century AD) writings.

The use of saffron as a natural dye was fairly widespread in Arabia, Europe, Persia, and India. It was used to colour religious and royal garments. Saffron was considered the colour of renunciation in India, where its flowers were used to dye clothes. After the death of Buddha, his followers in Kashmir began using saffron to dye their clothes using a mixture of roots and tubers, plants, bark, leaves, flowers, and fruits. The colour was temporary, so Tibetan Buddhist monks were known to dye their robes each year.

The active ingredient for dyeing in saffron is crocin, which is extracted from the flower petals. Traditionally, forest monks wear ochre (obtained from jackfruit heartwood) robes and city monks wear saffron robes, though variations exist. Today, though, saffron has been replaced by turmeric, which is also yellow, but less expensive.

The Talmud contains multiple references to saffron, and it is one of the 11 ingredients of the Ketoret Holy Incense. In Christianity, saffron is not a spice of major religious significance. There is a single reference to saffron in the Bible in Song of Solomon 4:14, where it is mentioned along with other incenses. During the Crusades, Christians brought large quantities of saffron, a highly valued commodity then, from the Holy Land to their European homes in France, and England. Saffron was then extensively planted in France and England and became hugely popular.

In fifteenth century AD Germany, adulterating saffron was a crime punishable by burning at the stake. In England, royal ladies often wore saffron in their hair, a practice that was ultimately forbidden by Henry VIII. In Arabic, saffron is called *zafran,* and used extensively in food, and coffee. The Middle East is the biggest importer of saffron. Islam, however, forbids the wearing of saffron-coloured clothes by adult males (Wikipedia).

The plant has been used as medicine across all herbal medicinal systems. Traditionally, the species is used for stomach cramps, flatulence, respiratory ailments, blood disorders, heart diseases, and as an aphrodisiac. It is a folk remedy for headaches and colds, and has antidiarrheal, and antidysentery properties. It is useful in treating scanty menstruation, and poor seminal mobility.

Saffron is one of the 770 medicinal plants mentioned in the *Sushruta Samhita.* In Ayurveda, saffron is used to improve skin tone, and reduce acne in skin creams and herbal facial masks, as well as in wound healing. When mixed with sandalwood paste, it cools the skin. Mediterraneans and Mesopotamians associated saffron with fertility and sexual potency.

Hippocrates and Galen mention using saffron to improve digestion, reduce flatulence and colic, and calm the nerves of adults and children. Avicenna in Book II of *Canon of Medicine* (*al-Qanun fi al-tib*) describes various medicinal uses of saffron, including its use as an antidepressant, hypnotic, anti-inflammatory, hepatoprotective, bronchodilator, aphrodisiac, labour inducer, and emmenagogue. Most of these effects have been studied in modern pharmacology, and are well documented.

In Traditional Chinese Medicine, saffron is claimed to be useful in conditions related to the heart and liver. It is used to invigorate blood supply, release toxins, and relieve high fevers and related conditions caused by pathogenic heat. Saffron is also used as a herbal cure for cold and cough, and in dentistry. The pharmacological data on saffron and its constituents, including crocin, crocetin, and safranal, are similar to those found in Avicenna's monograph (Phytotherapy Research., 2013, Hosseinzadeh, Nassiri-Asl).

C. sativus is known to have antihypertensive, anticonvulsant, antitussive, antigenototoxic, antioxidant, cytotoxic, anxiolytic, antidepressant, aphrodisiac, antinociceptive, anti-inflammatory, and relaxant properties. Modaghegh et al. (2008) conducted trials on a sample of 10 people who were administered saffron tablets, and showed reduction in both high systolic and arterial blood pressure. It also improves memory, learning, and sleep, and increases blood flow in the retina and choroid. In high doses, it has a narcotic effect.

C. sativus may alleviate symptoms of premenstrual syndrome according to a 2008 study, published in the *British Journal of Obstetrics and Gynecology*. After taking *C. sativus* twice a day during two menstrual cycles, the experiment group showed great improvement in premenstrual symptoms, compared to those assigned a placebo. However, because it is used to break blood clots, those on blood thinning medications, or women who experience heavy menstruation, should avoid saffron altogether. A New York Langone Medical Centre publication states that trials to validate saffron's ability to treat depression indicate positive results. The plant also shows promise in the treatment of cancer, reduction of cholesterol, protection against side effects of cisplatin, and enhancement of mental function.

ONYCHA (GUM TRAGACANTH, BENZOIN, MOLLUSK, OR LABDANUM)

Onycha is one of the four spices mentioned in the Old Testament (Exodus 30:34), and as an ingredient of Ketoret. Like many other herbs and spices mentioned during Biblical times, the origin of onycha is shrouded in debate, starting with the name itself. In Greek, it means "fingernail." Various scholars have argued that the origins of onycha include one of the four following options: gum tragacanth from the Astralagus species; benzoin from the Styrax species; a mollusk; and the labdanum plant.

Gum tragacanth, a tree gum, has a resin that falls on the ground and looks like fingernails. It is used as an incense fixative. However, Hebrew literature does not support onycha as a tree-based resin. This book considers benzoin to be the spice stacte, from the Stryax species, and thus an unlikely candidate for onycha.

Some argue that onycha is the operculum (lid or cover) of a marine mollusk, such as *Strombus lentiginosus* from the Red Sea, or the Mediterranean Sea Snail. Nawata (1997) has done extensive historical and ethnographical studies on the operculum and gastropod trade in Sudan. He identified the ancient port town of Badi in South-eastern Sudan on the Red Sea as an important port town for trade with Asia, Africa, Egypt, and other Mediterranean powers.

Locally, opercula are called *Dufr*, or fingernails of the sea. The export of four species (*Strombus lentiginosus, Murex anguliferus, Onyx marinus,* and *Unguis odoratus*) remains a major source of income to local communities. Opercula are widely used as incense in Sudan. They are first washed with an alkali solution and then treated with alcohol, vinegar, and water. A similar process is followed in China and Japan, whereas other places soak the opercula in fermented berry juice or strong white wine. They are then heated in oil to draw out the incense, which collects as a residue in the oil.

The residue is used as a fixative. Powdered operculum is also added to incense sticks. Old Arabic medical books describe the use of operculum to cure stomach pains, liver illnesses, epilepsy, and regulation of the menstrual cycle (Levey, 1961; Ibn Masawaih and His Treatise on Simple Aromatic Substances: Studies in the History of Arabic Pharmacology I. J. Hist. Medicine & Allied Sci., 16: 407; Meyerhof and Sobhy, 1932).

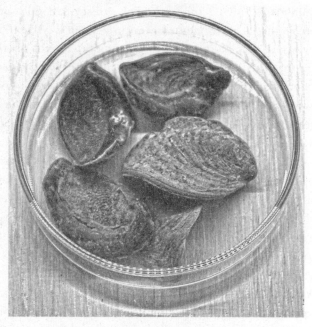

Figure 38 "Operculum of Mollusca, Jerusalem.
A Medical Diagnosis Exhibition IMG 9776" by Deror

However, the Talmud specifically states that onycha came from a plant, not a tree or animal. Other Jewish texts indicate that onycha was a resin exudate, pointing again to a non-animal origin. Furthermore, Jews considered fish and water animals to be unclean. Thus, the final candidate for onycha is labdanum. Labdanum can be *Cistus ladanifer* and *Cistus creticus*, which are both called rock rose or rose of Sharon. The leaves and twigs exude a musky-sweet, sticky, brown resin that is high in waxes. The name rose of Sharon perhaps comes from the fact that the plant grows extensively on the Israeli Sharon plains, which lie between Jaffa and Mount Carmel. The plant is native to the western Mediterranean region, where it thrives in the hot summers and cool dry winters, grows to 2.5 metres, and is cultivated for its scented foliage, and showy flowers. The plant is a vigorous, dense, upright shrub, covered with an aromatic resin exudate and bears ornamental white flowers.

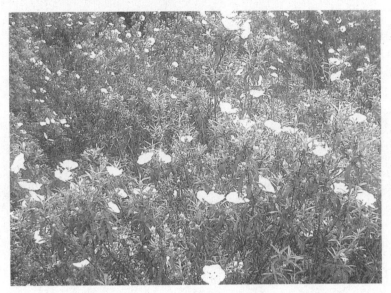

Figure 39 Cistus ladanifer in Spain, "Jaral2" by Javier martin, own work

According to Pliny the Elder, a herb called *ladan* (which is Arabic for labdanum) had a fragrant smell. The Bible mentions rose of Sharon: "I am the rose of Sharon, and the lily of the valleys. As the lily among thorns, so is my love among the daughters. As the apple tree among the trees of the wood, so is my beloved among the sons. I sat down under his shadow with great delight, and his fruit was sweet to my taste" (Song of Solomon 2 King James Version).

Egyptian pharaohs used the resin to apply artificial beards made from goat hair, which was a popular fashion among the elite. The resin was collected with a claw-like comb from the coats of animals who wandered around the shrubs and collected the gum in their hair. Herodotus mentions this in *Historia Book Thalia:*

Ledanum, which the Arabs call ladanum, is procured in a yet stranger fashion. Found in a most inodorous place, it is the sweetest-scented of all substances. It is gathered from the beards of he-goats, where it is found sticking like gum, having come from the bushes in which they browse. It is used in many types of unguents, and is what the Arabs burn chiefly as incense. Concerning the spices of Arabia, let no more be said. The whole country is scented with them, and exhales an odour marvellously sweet.

Most modern labdanum is from Spain. The oleoresin is collected directly from the plant and then steam distilled to yield the orange-brown essential oil. The yields of oil are very low, just 0.1 percent. In the early part of the twentieth century, a large rake called a ladanisterion was used to collect the oleoresin. The ladanisterion had leather strips to whip the leaves. The resinous sap that exuded from the damaged leaves adhered to the leather and was scraped off with a knife, and then formed into bars or balls. Harvesting today is also done manually with the help of a sickle.

Labdanum has two forms: cistus concrete, a dark brown mass, and cistus absolute, a highly viscous liquid. Cistus concrete is produced from the plant's aerial parts with the help of an extraction solvent that is eliminated during the concentration process. Cistus absolute is produced by washing the cistus concrete with ethanol. Glazing and filtration help rid the resin of waxes. Cistus concrete yields about 65 percent cistus absolute. Both cistus concrete and absolute are used in manufacturer of fragrances.

Labdanum oil (or cistus oil) is an important fixative in perfume. It is prized for its vegetal mossy aroma, and provides leather, musk oil, and ambergris notes. Its ambergris scent is especially valuable, since ambergris is now banned, as it is derived from the endangered sperm whale. The scent is said to retrieve subconscious memories, feelings, and moods.

Labdanum strengthens the body and provides warmth and sensuality. It is also considered useful in skincare preparations, especially for mature skin and wrinkles. It mixes well with amber, bay laurel, calamus, cardamom, chamomile, copal-black, iris root, lavender, musk seed, nutmeg, oakmoss, opopanax, patchouli, rosemary, rose, saffron, sandalwood, spikenard, storax, tolu balsam, and turmeric.

The Japanese use labdanum in their traditional Neriko incense mixtures that were used to scent the sleeves of traditional Japanese dresses worn in tea, and other ceremonial occasions. Labdanum is regarded as a spiritual or meditation oil. The oil was mixed with aromas of cypress patchouli and other oriental oils. Elizabethan pomanders contained labdanum as an ingredient.

Labdanum's traditional medicinal properties have been studied and validated in scientific studies. For example, the species was observed to reduce proliferation of Candida, *S. aureus*, and *E. coli* (Barrajon-Catalan et al 2010). It is regarded as a restorative, tonic, astringent, wound healer, and emmenagogue. Traditionally, the gum was used to treat diarrhoea, dysentery, catarrh, and menstrual disorders.

COSTUS

Costus comes from the root of plants in the Saussurea genus that grow in the higher elevations of the Himalayas in Asia, Tibet, and China. The name costus means "coming from the East" in Greek. The rhizome is cut, dried, and exported. Costus is rich in resinoids, inulin, alkaloids, tannins and sugars. Sesquiterpene lactones have been reported to be the major phytochemicals of this species.

Costus root is burnt in shrines or used as a tonic in hot baths. Smaller pieces are ground into powder and used to make incense sticks, including joss sticks. An essential oil is extracted by steam distillation from the root. In undiluted form, the oil is thick and difficult to use. Costus essential oil has an aroma often described as human hair, fur, or wet dog. As it ages, it develops a sweeter aroma with rosy undertones. It blends well with sandalwood, vetiver, rose, violet, patchouli, and floral fragrances like ylang ylang, patchouli, opopanax, and myrrh.

Costus root oil has been used in massage oils, body fragrances, laundry detergents, air fresheners, perfumes, diffusers, bath oils, soaps, and hair treatments. Ancient cloth merchants used costus oil to protect valuable silks and textiles from moths. However, it is a dermal irritant, and should not be applied directly to the skin. Thus, costus perfumes have been largely replaced with synthetics.

Costus is one of the 11 ingredients in the Ketoret incense mentioned in the Talmud. The Romans used it both as a culinary spice and perfume. Theophrastus listed it as one of the principal plants in perfumes of the time. Pliny mentions two varieties of costus, a white and black variety. The white variety was considered more fragrant, and came from an Arabic plant, *Costus speciosus syn C Arabica*. The root, which is the source of incense, is yellow, and the bark is white. It is said that the Hellenist King Seleucus Callinicus (c. 246 BC) sent costus imported from India as a gift to the Milesian King. According to Pliny, the price of costus was around 5 denarii per pound.

Waly (2009) has argued that *Costus spicatus* is actually *Saussurea lappa*. Saussurea is a Eurasian genus with 300 species, of which 61 are found in the high-altitude Himalayan regions of India and the rest in cooler regions of the Arctic, Asia, and North America. *S. lappa* is a perennial shrub often found as an understorey in birch forests. The plants can grow to a height of 3 metres. It is one of the most common members of the species, and was a major spice export to ancient Rome (Wikipedia). Its root has a bitter and acrid taste.

It is known as *Qust* in Arabic, and was used at the time of the Prophet Mohammed as a medicine, and post-menstrual wash. Oil prepared with *Qust* and olive oil was said to be effective as a muscle toner and as a treatment for alopecia and chloasma. With vinegar, it is effective in treating ringworm infections. The root was also used to treat toothache, asthma, dysentery, skin diseases, and rheumatism. In the *Hadith Mustadrak-al-Hakim*, narrated by Jabir Bin Abdullah, the Prophet stated, "If someone's child gets Azra or headache then she should take Qust and after grinding it in water, apply it to the child." *Azra* is an ancient term used in Arabia. It might be interpreted as tonsillitis.

The plant has been extensively cultivated since the 1920s in the high-altitude Lahaul valleys of Himachal Pradesh in the Himalayan state of India, in Kashmir, and in the Garhwal region in the hill state of Uttarakhand, in the northern part of India. It is regarded locally as green gold, and is a major non-timber forest product, and an important source of income for locals, who also smoke the leaves with tobacco.

There is a huge demand for the essential oil, known in India as *kuth*, and the herbal industry in India is the major consumer of most output. The Indian government requires a permit to export *kuth* roots. Efforts to encourage cultivation of *S. lappa* by local communities in India have been unsuccessful, mainly because of a lack of understanding of the business dynamics surrounding regulation, and a low return of investment. There are reports that the traditional cultivators of *kuth* have replaced it with potato, and other more profitable crops.

The Convention on International Trade in Endangered Species of Wild Fauna and Flora (2009) estimates that *kuth* root exports from India were 10,000 kilograms, mostly to Europe, Japan, and the Middle East. The Convention (2007) also estimates that root imports from China were 16,280 kilograms. High demand has led to over-exploitation of the plant. Thus, it was placed on the critical endangered species as *S. costus* in 1975, then as *S. lappa* in 1985 (Convention on International Trade in Endangered Species of Wild Fauna and Flora, 2011). It is an expensive product, and adulteration is common. The aromatic root of *Inula racemosa* from the Himalayan region is often used as an adulterant of costus root, and vetiver oil is an adulterant in costus root oil.

In Ayurveda, *kushta* (costus) is an ancient *rasayana* (medication) mentioned in the Atharvaveda as a remedy for excess *jvara* (fever). *Kushta* was considered a divine plant, derived from heavenly sources, because it grows high in the Himalayas. It was considered to be the brother of the divine *soma*, a psychedelic plant consumed by ancient Aryans for strength in battle. Some regard soma to be a mythical plant; others claim it is extinct. Its habitat was probably the central Asian region around Lake Balkash from where the Aryans are said to have migrated to India and Persia (Cairae, *An Aryan Journey*).

It helps normalise and strengthen digestion, detoxify, enhance fertility, and reduce pain. Many Ayurvedic medicines manufactured in India contain *kushta* root, which is believed to possess antiseptic and anti-inflammatory properties. Unani recognises costus as a great medicinal plant with carminative, aphrodisiac, and anthelmintic effects. It was also thought to be a brain stimulant, and a treatment for liver diseases, deafness, headache, paralysis, cough, fever, inflammation, and ophthalmic conditions (Madhuri et al., 2012). The essential oil of the root is believed to relax bronchial muscles, providing relief in cases of bronchitis, and asthma.

Saussurea costus root is one of 50 fundamental medicinal herbs in Traditional Chinese Medicine. It can move qi, relieve pain, fortify the spleen, and disperse food (Jiaju Zhou et al., 2010). It is antiseptic and is traditionally used to treat digestive and respiratory system ailments. Costus oil is also useful in treating nematode infections.

According to Waly (2009), *S. lappa* might be used in phlegmatic diseases. It is effective in treating general weakness from diarrhoea and cholera. It can be used on clothes to repel insects. Internally, it is a good expectorant, antispasmodic, and neurotoxin that can treat cough, bronchitis, bronchial asthma, paralysis, facial palsy, and neurasthenia.

The root's anticonvulsant properties have been studied and results validated on experiments on rats (Ambavade et al 2009). Different pharmacological in vitro, and in vivo models have convincingly demonstrated the ability of *S. costus* to exhibit anti-inflammatory, anti-ulcer, anticancer, and hepatoprotective properties. Several molecules isolated from this plant have potential as bioactive molecules (Pandey et al., 2007).

A number of scientific experiments, including human trials, validate some of the traditional medicinal uses of the root. Experiments on rats indicate cardioprotective properties of the root. It is mandatory to follow drug discovery protocols before any use of the root and essential oil can be unambiguously stated (Ambawade et al., 2009; Hasson et al., 2013; Kim et al., 2014).

HENNA

Lawsonia inermis is the botanical name for henna. This small tree grows to a height of 5–7 metres. The plant prefers a dry and hot climate. It grows extensively in the Mediterranean region, Egypt, neighboring countries of Northern and Eastern Africa, the Arabian Peninsula, parts of Australasia, and Southern Asia.

When frequently clipped, leaf formation increases, thus it is a popular hedge plant for property demarcation, because the hedges become impenetrable to animals, and cattle prefer not to graze on the leaves. The best dye yield is obtained from leaves when air temperatures are between 35–45 degrees Celsius. Leaves of henna are plucked, dried, packed, and then sold.

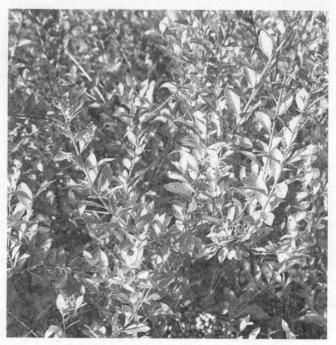

Figure 40 "Lawsonia inermis (Mehndi) in Hyderabad,
AP W IMG 0527" by J.M. Garg, own work

The FAO estimates the global trade in henna leaves and powder to be 9,000 metric tonnes. The major suppliers of henna are India, Pakistan, Iran, and Sudan. Many Middle Eastern countries produce henna, but also import substantial quantities to meet high demand. The major importers are Islamic countries in the Middle East and Northern Africa.

Europe and North America are significant, but much smaller, markets. Saudi Arabia is the largest importer (3,000 metric tonnes). In Europe, the biggest importer is France (250 metric tonnes), followed by the United Kingdom and Germany. In the Muslim world, the henna trade is driven by religious customs, as well as preference for modern cosmetics and fashion. Much of the export to Europe and North America is driven by the trend towards natural products.

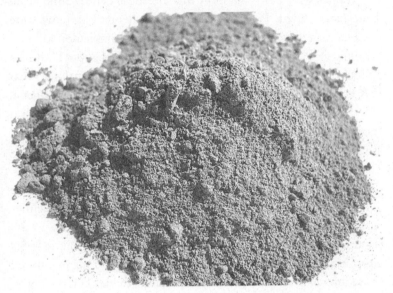

Figure 41 Henna powder, "Henna for hair"

Since the first millennium BC, when henna was closely associated with the divine coupling of goddess and consort in Canaanite Israel, henna has been associated with beauty, love, and eroticism. The earliest reference to henna is at a site discovered in Catal Huyuk, Turkey, that dates back to the Neolithic period in the seventh millennium BC. It shows henna being used to decorate hands, and perhaps links henna to the fertility goddess.

Mummified bodies from about 3400 BC in Egypt show henna-dyed hair and fingers. The mummy of Ramses II (c. 1279–1213 BC) has hennaed fingertips and toes. Excavations in Jericho show that henna was used to dye hair as far back as 1900–1500 BC. Several statues in Italy from the fourth and third centuries BC depict women with hennaed hair. Dioscorides notes that crushed leaves were used to dye hair orange and a plaster made from henna leaves was effective to treat inflammations and blisters.

Writings by Pliny mention that the best henna came from Israel, and Egypt. Perfumes made from henna blossoms were used at that time. According to a Jewish compilation of oral rabbinic legal traditions codified in Israel around 200 AD, henna was an important agricultural commodity and medicinal herb that was taxed by the state. In his botanical work *Peri Photon Historias* (*Concerning the Investigation of Plants*), Theophrastus describes an incense preparation of henna, and other spices like cardamom, for use in scented wine.

Henna is also mentioned extensively in the Islamic hadiths. The Prophet Muhammad preferred its scent. Hadiths prescribe rules for adorning man, woman, and a person who is neither male nor female, with henna. Colouring hair with henna is still regarded by many Muslims as an act of love for God, and his Prophet. Henna perfumes remain popular and are manufactured in traditional perfume centres in India and Arabia. The Bible also associates henna with beauty, as in Song of Songs 1:14.

Henna is used to dye cotton, silk, and other natural fibres, as well as leather, and leather products. The dye is temporary. In India, henna is used for body art during festivals and celebrations, including extensive use in bridal makeup in Southern Asia and the Middle East. In rural areas and in traditional families, the application of henna to a bride is accompanied by dance, song, and music. Beautiful patterns of flowers, leaves, and other complex artistic patterns are drawn on the hands, feet, and the other body parts by artists who use a nozzle-based instrument to apply the henna paste. The paste dries for a couple hours before it is washed off, leaving reddish orange imprints on the body. The staining is attributed to lawsone, an active ingredient that reacts with skin proteins to create a reddish orange stain. Lawsone is released only when it interacts with an acidic solution like lemon juice or tea leaves. Fresh henna leaves, if ground to paste and applied as such, do not yield a dye.

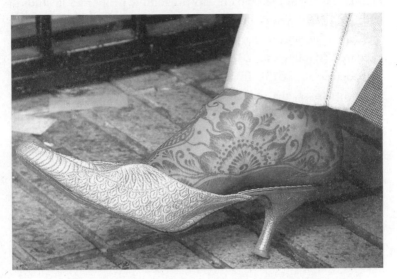

Figure 42 "Henna on foot in Morocco" by Bjørn Christian Tørrissen, own work by uploader, http://bjornfree.com/galleries.html

Henna body art has acquired global popularity, and exports of henna powder to Europe and North America have increased substantially. The U.S. FDA does not ban the use of henna as hair dye, but it has not approved its use for direct contact with skin. A 2013 study commissioned by the European Union, and conducted by the Scientific Committee on Consumer Safety, concluded that lawsone is safe in hair dye. The traditional use of henna as a perfume is now limited to the preparation of Indian or Middle Eastern perfume called *attar*, which is mixed with sandalwood.

In his work *Naturalis Historia*, Pliny the Elder mentions a green ointment with henna that was used to treat sores on the head and in the mouth. A compress of the henna leaves is said to be good for burns and sprains.

More recently, henna leaves have been observed to be an effective antibacterial against *E. coli* (Abulyazid et al., 2013). Henna leaves have shown chemo-preventive properties in studies with rats. The wound-healing property, as observed in ancient medicinal literature, was also studied in rats and appears to be validated (Babili et al., 2013; Chandra Kalyan Reddy et al., 2011; Kapadia et al., 2013). In tribal regions of Eastern India in the State of Orissa, the indigenous people use henna leaves to treat liver ailments. This property was studied in rats and findings were positive (Hossein et al., 2011).

CHAPTER 4

SACRED
TREES

～◆～

Ancient civilisations and religious texts of all three
religions of the Biblical lands (Christianity, Jewish,
and Islam) have attributed immense importance to
trees, which were valued for food, animal feed, oil,
fuel, and construction. This section describes seven
sacred trees mentioned in the Bible: cedar, date palm,
sycamore, olive, pomegranate, willow, and myrtle.
Ancient Egyptians associated trees with the afterlife,
and with their popular deities. For example, Horus was
associated with the acacia. The Egyptian *Book of the
Dead* mentions that two sycamore, or *nehet*, trees stood
at the eastern gate of heaven from where the sun god
Ra emerged each morning. The tree is regarded as a
manifestation of the goddess Nut, Isis, and Hathor.
Sycamore trees were often planted in cemeteries, and
coffins made from sycamore wood helped lead the
dead person to the mother tree goddess.

Myrrh trees were also sacred and were planted on the the terraces of the Funerary Temple of Hatshepsut at Deir el-Bahari (c. 1480 BC). This temple is dedicated to the Egyptian sun god Amon Ra, and can still be seen in the Valley of the Kings in Egypt. A date palm branch was the symbol of the god Heh, who represented eternity.

The willow was considered sacred to the Egyptian god of the afterlife, Osiris. Just as Hindu tradition in India claims that the Hindu gods sought shelter in *Ficus religiosa*, ancient Egyptian tradition claims that Osiris's body was sheltered by a willow after he was killed. It is believed that his body was dismembered and buried in tombs throughout Egypt, where willow then grew.

In ancient Greece, the oak tree was sacred to Zeus, and the myrtle tree to Aphrodite. A sacred olive tree is said to have stood in the Pandrosium near the Erechtheum Temple (421–405 BC) on the Acropolis. Ancient Greek literature contains multiple references to sacred groves. In Greek myths, the spirits of trees are personified in female form. In ancient Rome, a fig tree sacred to Romulus grew near the Forum, along with multiple sacred groves throughout the city.

Trees were important in the ancient Canaanite religion that pre-dates the Hebrew Bible. Canaanites lived in what is now Lebanon and Syria. The Bible mentions the Canaanites and the sacredness of the trees: "Abram passed through the land as far as the site of Shechem, to the oak of Moreh. Now the Canaanite was then in the land" (Genesis 12:6). In the Canaanite religion, Asherah was perhaps a fertility goddess, and consort of the pagan god Baal. In the Greek and Latin translations of the Bible, *asherah* is interpreted as "grove" or "wood." In the early years of the Hebrew people, Asherah was represented in Jewish temples in the form of a wooden pole or tree, planted next to the Jewish god YHWH. It is believed that YHWH appeared to Abraham while he prayed beneath a terebinth tree. A descendant of this tree is venerated by pilgrims and visitors to Hebron.[1]

References to the bounty of God in the form of trees and plants are also made in the Koran. Koran Sura references fruit, and other plants as gifts from God: "It is He who sends down water from the sky with which We bring forth the buds of every plant. From these We bring forth green foliage and close-growing grain, palm-trees laden with clusters of dates, vineyards and olive groves, and pomegranates alike and different. Behold their fruits when they ripen. Surely in these there are signs for true believers" (Al-An'_ am 6:99).

Although tree worship is denounced in the Bible as idol worship (Deuteronomy 12:2), trees were immensely important to the people of these regions. The Bible contains more than 525 plant references, including 22 trees (e.g., acacia, almond, apple, carob, cypress, date palm, ebony, fig, oak, pine, pistachio, poplar, pomegranate, frankincense, lign aloe, sycamore fig, plane, tamarisk, terebinth, thyme, walnut, and willow).

Some, like palm and olive, have been associated with worship, or actively used in the Jewish temple. Others, like the willow, are mentioned in 25 verses of *the Bible*. Fruit trees such as the date palm, fig, olive, pomegranate, and tamarisk were afforded protection in Deuteronomy 20:19–20. Fruit trees are described as a gift from God in Genesis 1:29. When the Jews were exiled from Egypt and came to the Holy Land, they used trees for food, shade, timber, and oil.

---

[1] A similar, though probably historically unrelated, ritual is still practiced in India today. Every year, the local people select and cut the best tree with the cleanest bole to plant in their temple. This celebratory ritual is, mercifully, now on the decline. While there is no connection between Asherah and this Hindu practice, this shows common beliefs among ancient cultures and religions.

The ancient Greek, Sumerian, Babylonian, and pagan religions, influenced the people of these lands, and elements of some pagan traditions have survived. For example, the gold candelabra featured in Jewish temples depict the almond tree, and Jews valued pistachio, cedar, and sycamore trees. Cedars still grow in the highlands, and sycamore in the lowlands of Israel and surrounding areas. Some scholars argue that the Tree of Life, and Tree of Knowledge of Good and Evil in the Garden of Eden (Genesis 2:9) represent this view.

The meaning of the Tree of Life varies with the culture and identity of the people. For example, the Druids believed that the tree of life was oak, a long-lived tree that hosts mistletoe, their most sacred plant. The ancient Jews believed it was cedar, which provided wood and precious aromatic oil. The Assyrians believed it was the date tree, which produced food and date wine (a libation of the gods), and symbolised the bridge between the world and God, and his heaven.

Six trees are especially important in the Bible, and are associated with Genesis: the Tree of Life, the Tree of the Knowledge of Good and Evil, fruit-bearing trees, the prophet's oak at Mamre, the components of Noah's ark, and the date palm. In the Christian church, the Tree of Life is the pole on which Jesus was crucified, and died. It is believed to be the sycamore, which is mentioned multiple times in the Scriptures.

The botanical species of the Tree of Knowledge of Good and Evil remains elusive, though the baobab tree is mentioned as one of the trees that Abraham's ancestors valued for its bark, leaves, and fruit. The baobab tree also stores water in its thick corky stem, and is a source of drinking water, particularly during dry months. The correct scientific and botanical name for the oak at Mamre remains elusive, just as in the case of many plants mentioned in the Bible.

The contents of Noah's Ark are shrouded in mystery. Traditionally, the ark contained samples of living creatures from the time of the Great Flood. However, there are no scientific evidence regarding these claims.

The date palm is among the most prized trees of the Middle East, North Africa, and the Mediterranean region. It is a source of food, and was also used in construction in the second and first millennium BC. Other fruit trees include the pomegranate, and pistachio. The cyclical regeneration of trees represented the cycle of life and death, as demonstrated in the following verse:

> The LORD God planted a garden toward the east, in Eden; and there He placed the man whom He had formed. Out of the ground the LORD God caused to grow every tree that is pleasing to the sight and good for food; the tree of life also in the midst of the garden, and the tree of the knowledge of good and evil. Now a river flowed out of Eden to water the garden; and from there it divided and became four rivers . . ." (Genesis 2:8–9)

CEDAR

Cedar is a broad term that could represent a range of genera and species found in different parts of the world. Some popular genera of cedar trees include Cedrus, Cupressus, Juniperus, and Widdringtonia. Cedar grows extensively in the cool temperate regions of Asia, Middle East, Europe, and North America. *Cedrus libani,* or Lebanese cedar was a popular cedar species of the Mediterranean, used extensively as a source of timber and oil..

The earliest archaeological evidence of cedar use dates back to the Bronze Age in the fourteenth century BC. Resinous woods were in great demand in antiquity, mostly for construction and shipbuilding across Mesopotamia, Persia, Turkey, Rome, Greece, Egypt, and Israel. The first Muslim fleet (c. 645 AD) was purportedly built using timber from the region. A shipwreck discovered near the city of Uluburum in Turkey was made from cedar.

During the Crusades, Cedar was used in shipbuilding, and for building Umayyad palaces, mosques, and other construction in the Mediterranean and Mesopotamian regions. King Solomon contracted King Hiram of Tyre to extract cedar logs from the mountains of Lebanon to build the temple at Jerusalem (He 2 Samuel 7:1–2; 2 Samuel 5:11; 1 Kings 5:6).

Lebanese cedar was used in the timber-scarce societies of Egypt, Palestine, Greece, and the Roman Empire. Cedars are widely dispersed in Asia, Europe, and North America and the cedar forests of Lebanon are mentioned often in the Bible. The Old and the New Testament contain multiple references to cedar, mostly as construction timber. Most of the cedar forests of Lebanon that contain *Cedrus libani* have disappeared, except for a few stands on the mountain slopes.

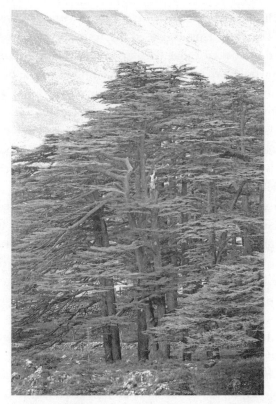

Figure 43 Lebanon cedar trees, "Cedars02" by Jerzy Strzelecki, own work

Cedar grows abundantly in the northwestern region of North America, and was one of the most important Native American ceremonial plants. Many tribes used it as incense and a purifying herb. Cedar was associated with prayer, healing, dreams, and protection against disease. This view is synonymous with the views expressed in the Bible (Leviticus 14:1–7, 33–53). It describes a house-cleaning process that uses two live clean birds, cedar, scarlet yarn, and hyssop.

Cedar was also prized for its aroma, and cedar oil was particularly valued in Babylon and Egypt. A clay tablet from Egypt

(c. 1800 BC) describes an order to import oils of cedar, myrrh, and cypress. The Egyptians also used the resin to mummify bodies. Initially, they soaked cedar bark in olive oil after grinding it. In this oil, a wool cloth was then soaked and burnt. The heat pulled the essential oil out of the bark and into the olive oil. When the wool cloth was squeezed, it released the essential oil.

Greek physicians used resin and tar to make cough medicines and salves for external use. The ancient Sumerians made a blue pigment by grinding cedar oil and cobalt compounds in a mortar and pestle.

Overexploitation was evident even in ancient times. In the Epic of Gilgamesh, when Gilgamesh seized the axe and felled the cedar, Humbaba heard the noise far away and was enraged. He cried out, "Who is this that violated my woods and cut down my cedar?" Roman Emperor Hadrian declared the cedar forests to be imperial property, perhaps to keep the cedar trees for exclusive state use.

The Bible mentions cedar (2 Kings 19:23; Isaiah 41:19; Zechariah 11:2). The Phoenicians, who controlled the ports of Tyre, Sidon, and others along the Mediterranean Sea coast, had a near monopoly over the lumber business. Cedar is a slow-growing species, and principles of scientific forest management that ensure sustainable logging had not yet been developed. As a result, the cedar trees of Lebanon, the best in the region, were nearly destroyed.

After the forests of Lebanon, the next source of lumber was Amanus (now in southern Turkey), which was part of the Greek empire (Meiggs, 1984, p. 62). Around the time of Plato, the local forests of Greece were denuded of cedar, so Athenians imported lumber from Phoenicia in substantial quantities (Semple, 1931, p. 276).

Today, most cedar oil is from cypresses and junipers, and most global production occurs in North America and China. Very little oil is produced from the true cedars of the Cedrus genus. The following table lists the major cedar oil species, based on FAO data:

Family Pinaceae	
Cedrus deodara (Roxb.) Loud.	Himalayan cedar wood,
Cedrus atlantica Manetti	deodar Atlas cedar wood
Family Cupressaceae	
Cupressus funebris Endl.	Chinese cedar wood
Juniperus virginiana L.	Virginia cedar wood, eastern red cedar
Juniperus mexicana Schiede or *Juniperus ashei Buch*, according to Adams (1987)	Texas cedar wood
Juniperus procera Hochst	East African cedar wood
Widdringtonia whytei Rendle	Mulanje cedar wood

Excluding the People's Republic of China, whose magnitude of consumption of domestically produced cedar oil is not known, the United States, Europe, and Japan are the major markets for the oil. The United States and China are the two major producers and exporters of cedar oil and their derivative products.

Most American cedar oil production is derived from the invasive juniper species that is a waste wood from the timber industry. Essential oil yield from North American cedars can reach 3.8 percent. The United States consumes much of its own Texas and Virginia cedar oils, but it also imports significant quantities of Chinese oil.

In 1995, the production of cedar wood oil in the United States was estimated at 1,640 metric tonnes, and the FAO estimated annual imports in the range of 300 to 400 metric tonnes. Japanese imports have averaged around 170 metric tonnes, with most of it coming from the United States.

Europe prefers Chinese oil, which has a lower cedrol content, thinner texture, and stronger fragrance compared to American oil. The antiseptic properties of cedar oil are from the presence of the alkaloid cedrol. The average cedrol content is 25–42 percent in North American cedar and 8 percent in Chinese oil.

Eastern Africa used to be an important source of cedar oil, but overexploitation has substantially depleted the forests. In India, *Cedrus deodara* is sometimes used to produce oil. However, most of its production is domestically consumed, and there is no industrial production. Wooden railroad sleepers used to be made from *C. deodara* from the Himalayan region of India.

The modern process of creosoting (Semple, 1931, p. 282), in which the pine extract turpentine is used to seal wood, was used in India until a few decades ago, before concrete sleepers replaced wooden ones. The pine extract was also an ingredient in volatile oils, salves, and ointments. In Russia, oil is extracted from the Siberian pine *Pinus sibirica* by distilling the wood chips in water. After processing, derivatives, and their formulated products have a more diverse range of markets.

Cedar oil is widely used in the fragrance industry in soaps, air fresheners, floor polishes, and sanitation supplies. It is common to use the oil in deodorants, insecticides, mothproof bags, and other products. It is also an ingredient in well-known perfumes, such as Obsession, Chanel No. 5, Giorgio, Lauren, and Poison, and men's fragrances like Old Spice, Chaz, and English Leather.

The insecticidal and fungicidal properties of cedar oil have been widely recognised since ancient times. Hudson et al. (2011) showed that cedar oil was an effective decontamination agent for buildings. While the oil is used as an insect repellent in sprays and candles, direct application can irritate the skin. Pregnant women should not use the oil. If ingested, it can cause vomiting, and extensive damage to the digestive system.

The antiseptic, antimicrobial, antispasmodic, and antifungal properties of cedar have been studied and validated. Traditionally, the oil of cedar was used to relieve respiratory ailments, and studies have indicated that the oil has mucolytic properties. The oil is useful in treating skin ailments like acne, and seborrhea. Aromatherapy, with cedar oil, is used to provide relief in cases of arthritic pain, nervous tension, and anxiety.

It blends well with bergamot, benzoin, cinnamon, frankincense, juniper, jasmine, lemon, lime, lavender, rose, neroli, and rosemary. In Ayurvedic medicine, cedar leaves are used to treat tuberculosis. A decoction made from the heartwood treats chest infections, insomnia, and diabetes. The oil is also prescribed for syphilis and leprosy.

DATE PALM

Phoenix dactylifera, the date palm, or *tamar*, is a monocot plant from the Arecaceae family. The species is widely distributed in the East from the Indian subcontinent, and onto the Arabian Peninsula, the Mesopotamian and region of the Levant, to North Africa.

The tree often grows to a height of 25 metres. The treetop has a relatively small crown unlike branched dicotyledonous species. However, the fronds (leaves) of the tree are large, and offer good shade. The tree resists hot desert winds, but does require sufficient ground moisture to yield fruit.

Date palm (*Phoenix dactylifera* L.) is a high-energy crop, and one of the most nutritious fruits in the tropics and subtropics. It is rich in sugars, palmitic and organic acids, linoleic, lauric, myristic, and other fatty acids, vitamins A, B1, B2, and traces of vitamin C, niacin, potassium, calcium, iron, magnesium sulfur, phosphorus, chlorine, copper, and beta D glucan, a dietary fibre. Dates are a good source of phytochemicals like phenols, and carotenoids.

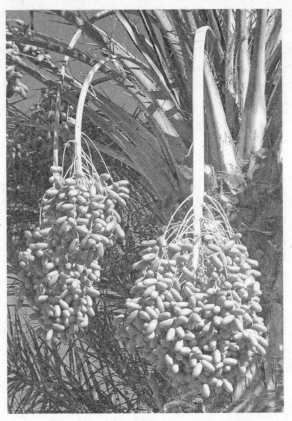

Figure 44 Date Palm tree with dates, "Dates on date palm"

Fossil records of date palm trees date back at least fifty million years. Some claim that date palm originates from the Indus Valley, because *Phoenix sylvestris*, the wild variety of date, and in all probability the predecessor of the date palm *Phoenix dactylifera*, still grows in India and Pakistan.

It is claimed that the species spread to Mesopotamia and the Red Sea region via traders, because of its value as a food source. It was cultivated from Northern Africa to India, and across the Biblical lands. Archaeological evidence indicates that cultivation of the palm occurred during the Neolithic era in Mehrgarh in modern Pakistan (c. 7000 BC), in Eastern Arabia (c. 6000 BC), and in the Harappan Indus and Sumerian regions (c. 2800–1800 BC).

Because date palms are found around oases in the desert regions of these territories, they came to symbolise immortality, longevity, and renewal. The date palm was cultivated mainly for its fruit, which could be eaten, fresh or dried. Wilkinson (1854) lists 360 date palm products. Popenoe 1913 lists and describes 1,500 cultivars of date palm.

The date fruit matures in about 200 days, in four stages. The first stage is *kimri*, or the unripe stage. The second stage is *khalal*, or the crunchy stage, at which point the fruit reaches full size. The third stage is *rutab*, or the ripe and soft stage. The final stage is *tamr*, which is the fully ripe and sun-dried stage. The fruit is harvested in the last three phases. Mature palms can produce 70 to 200 kilograms of dates per harvest season. Thinning of the date bunch allows space for new growth.

The Epic of Gilgamesh mentions date palm groves in the Tigris and Euphrates valleys in modern Iraq. The Code of Hammurabi (c. 1750 BC) notes that the date palm was worth double the price of the ground it occupies. The date palm was linked in ancient Egypt to the sun-bird, hence the genus name Phoenix.

Dates store well, which was useful in the desert climate of Egypt. Ancient Egyptians made date palm wine, and their priests wore sandals made from palm leaf. The tree was used to construct the temple of the moon god near Ur, regarded as the oldest city in Mesopotamia. Date palm fronds were used as thatching for roofs and baskets, and the trunks were used as supports in construction and plumbing. This low-quality wood remains an inexpensive option even today.

Date palm is associated with Egyptian gods Ammon Ra and Hathor, the goddess of love, fertility, music, and joy: "In a clean place shall I sit on the ground. Beneath the foliage of a date palm of the goddess Hathor . . ." (The Egyptian *Book of the Dead*). Excavations in Egypt have revealed images of a kneeling man holding a bunch of palm leaves. Scholars interpret this as an expression of longevity.

When a pharaoh celebrated the thirtieth jubilee of his reign, he held a bunch of palm leaves at mid-rib level during the Heb Sed ceremony. It was believed that the gods had carved notches into the mid-ribs that corresponded to the number of years left of the reign and life of the king (Nazir, 1970; Bircher, 1990). Palm groves were planted around monasteries in the Egyptian deserts, a practice still used today.

Date seeds have been found in the Kharga Oasis in the Libyan Desert area of Egypt. A mummy robed with date palm leaves dates to about 3500 BC (Bircher, 1990). A vat containing a beer cocktail using date palm was excavated in Hierakonpolis (Egypt), and dates to about 3450 BC (Amer, 1994). In the fifteenth century BC, date fruits were paid as wages for construction work at Dier El-Medina temple (Darby et al., 1977).

Date palm trees were cultivated in the gardens of nobles and kings. One gardener, whose garden was said to contain 170 date palm trees, covered the walls of his tomb with paintings of date palm trees. Date palm seeds were used as mortuary offerings in ancient Egypt. A number of excavations have uncovered date palm decorations that date as far back as third millennium BC. Rocky stones decorated with palm trees have been found in temples and tombs of the third and second millennium BC.

The ancient Greeks regarded palm as a sacred sign of Apollo. Cimon of Athens erected a bronze statue of a palm tree at Delphi, as part of a victory commemorating the Battle of Eurymedon (c. 469–466 BC; Wikipedia). In ancient Rome, palm was a symbol of champions and a palm branch was awarded to victors in athletic contests. The Romans considered dates a sweet delicacy, importing them from the Arabian Peninsula and Northern Africa.

Pliny stated that all the countries of the East made date palm wine. Palm leaves were considered sacred. They were used at ceremonial occasions like the anointment of a King. In the ancient Assyrian religion, the palm tree's crown represented heaven, and the base of the trunk represented earth. In ancient Mesopotamia, the date palm represented human fertility. In Africa, the date palm shape is said to be similar in shape to the female vagina.

According to Islam, date palm grows in the Garden of Paradise in heaven, and is regarded as a symbol of peace. Palm trees around oases were regarded as a gift of Allah. A *muezzin*, or crier, would climb a date palm tree to call the faithful to prayer. The Koran was apparently first written on palm leaves. There are multiple references to the date palm in the speeches and life of the Prophet Mohammed.

The first Islamic mosque, built in Madina after the death of the Prophet, was made from mud bricks and palm fronds, with columns made from palm trunks. The Prophet's burial place was decorated with palm sticks. It is said that, after the death of the Prophet Umar and Abu Bakr, the friends and close followers of the Prophet Mohammed ordered his scribe, Zayd Ibn Thabet, to collect and collate Koranic words written on the palm leaves. The written Koran probably was an outcome of these efforts.

Additionally, the Koran mentions the palm 20 times, 15 of which reference God's bounty to the human race. Some of these are included here:

It is He who sendeth down rain from the skies: with it We produce vegetation of all kinds: from some We produce green (crops), out of which We produce grain, heaped up (at harvest); Out of the date palm and its sheaths (or spathes) (come) clusters of dates hanging low and near. (An'âm, 99)

It is He who produceth gardens with trellises and without, and dates, and tilth with produce of all kinds and olives and pomegranates, similar (in kind) and different (in variety). (An'âm, 141)

Set forth to them the parable of two men: For one of them We provided two gardens of grape vines and surrounded them with date palms; in between the two We placed corn-fields. (Kahf, 32)

A good word like a goodly tree, whose root is firmly fixed, and its branches (reach) to the heavens. (Ibrahim, 24)

Annas said that the Prophet Mohammed said about this goodly tree that: This tree is the date palm tree. (El Nadawi, 1994)

In Judaism, date palm is called *tamar* and symbolises prosperity and abundance (Psalm 92:12). It is also a sign of joy and happiness. The frond of the date palm is part of the Jewish festival of Sukkot. Palm trees adorned ancient temples, and are described in Ezekiel (40:16), and other verses. When Jesus entered Jerusalem, his followers waved palm leaves in greeting. After Jesus' crucifixion, palm became a symbol of martyrdom for Christian people.

Today, the date belt stretches across the Indus Valley, Turkmenistan, and India in the east, to Somalia and Spain in the west. The FAO estimated the cultivation area for dates at 1.3 million ha in 2009 (FAO Statistics, 2010). The largest area (833,351 hectares) is in the Asian continent, and includes the Middle East. Africa cultivated 416,695 hectares of date palm, mostly in the north (392,200 hectares).

In the Americas and Europe, the production area is estimated at only a few thousand hectares. The 2009 worldwide production of dates was estimated at 7.3 million metric tonnes. In a decade, the production rose by more than one million metric tonnes. The production from Middle Eastern and Northern African countries was 2.7 million metric tonnes.

According to FAO statistics, the world's largest producer over the last five years has been Egypt, with an average production of 1.3 million metric tonnes, followed by Iran (just over 1 million metric tonnes), Saudi Arabia (979,017 metric tonnes), United Arab Emirates (754,400 metric tonnes), Pakistan (540,000 metric tonnes), Algeria (540,000 metric tonnes), and Sudan (333,500 metric tonnes). Other date-producing countries are Oman, Libya, Tunisia, Morocco, Yemen, Mauritania, Bahrain, Qatar, and Kuwait.

In terms of annual yields, the United States leads, with an estimated average of 6.7093 kg/ha. Next is Africa, especially the northern parts, producing 6.4974 kg/ha on average. In the Middle East, despite a large production area, yields are below the world average (5.3798 kg/ha).

With 70 percent sugar by weight, dates are referred to as natures' candy. Date palm is used as a sweetener, and fermented into vinegar and alcoholic beverages. A special type of date wine called *araqe* is still manufactured in rural Egypt. In India, a local wine is produced from date palm fruit. In times of drought and food scarcity, the trunk of the palm tree can be pulverised, and turned into an edible coarse flour.

Dry or soft dates are eaten raw, or used in cooking. The terminal bud is eaten as vegetable. In modern commercial production, the hard seed is mechanically separated from the sweet flesh. The fruit is then converted into cubes, pastes, spreads, and sugars. In areas where date palm is abundant, such as the Sahara, culled fruits are dehydrated, ground, and mixed with grain to produce a nutritious animal feedstock for camels, dogs, and horses. In many Arabic countries, dates are boiled in water to make a sweet tea.

The Bedouins, and other nomads of the desert boil milk with dates to make a sweet nutritious drink. Muslims traditionally break the Ramadan fast with dates.

Date palm trees are sometimes tapped to yield a sweet sap, which converts to sugar and alcohol in a few hours. Zahdi dates from Iraq produce good-quality, light-colored, dry wine. Date syrup makes a darker, sweeter wine. In India, date sugar is made from *Phoenix sylvestris*. Date seeds are also roasted, ground, and used to adulterate coffee, by unscrupulous people. *P. sylvestris* does not yield high-quality fruit, so it is tapped for a liquor called *toddy* by cutting the terminal bud, and collecting the sweet sap. Adding a small quantity of urea aids the fermentation process.

The ancient Egyptians used fresh dates, date kernels, dry myrrh, and wax, to form a paste to bandage swollen limbs. The Prophet Mohammed said that the direct external use of *tamr* paste cures the effects of poisonous bites. Eating ripe dates at bedtime was said to remove Ascaris worms.

Traditionally, dates are also used to treat liver ailments, hemorrhoids, and inflammation from kidney, cardiac, nervous, and other ailments. The pollen enhances fertility. Women use dates before, and after delivery, as a tonic for uterine muscles, to aid and prevent bleeding in childbirth, and as a lactagogue (the potassium, glycine, and threonine help activate the milk hormone prolactin). Dates are recommended in mouthwashes as a purgative, and the roots were used to relieve toothaches.

Ointments made from dates treat wounds and bruises. Dates also treat eye injuries, colds, fevers, cystitis, edema, sore throat, bronchial catarrh, liver cancer, low sperm count, and abdominal ailments. Combined with other herbs, they relieve swollen and aching legs, coughs, and sneezing. Dates are believed to fortify the body, enrich the blood, cure back pain, and invigorate the loins.

The sap from the leaves has been used as a remedy for nervousness and kidney problems. Date seeds were burnt to produce kohl for eyes. Date seed paste was found to relieve ague, and a paste of ripe dates in water acted as an antihistamine when applied externally to the skin. Its gum was used to treat diarrhea and counteract alcoholic intoxication.

Dates contain nutrients and minerals like potassium, copper, and magnesium, which have cardioprotective properties. Potassium reduces high blood pressure, and soluble fibre helps reduce cholesterol. The pollen, which yields an estrogenic principle, has shown a gonadotropic effect on young rats, perhaps explaining the traditional belief that dates possessed an aphrodisiac property when mixed with milk and cinnamon. Estron hormone is extracted from date seeds, and treated chemically to obtain stradiol, which is used in cancer treatments.

Al Qarawi et al. (2013) have shown that CCl4-induced liver damage in rats can be treated with date flesh or pit extract. Experiments conducted on rats indicate that antioxidants and fatty acids in *P. dactylifera* benefit the brain, although the psychological benefits are not clearly indicated (Ismail et al., 2013).

The oral administration of *P. dactylifera* extract along with a high-fat diet showed antihyperlipidemic efficacy of the species. Pujari et al. (2011) studied and validated its possible use in common carotid artery occlusion induced by oxidative stress and neuronal damage in rats.by

Hepatoprotective properties of date palm, along with *Glycyrrhiza glabra*, were studied and validated by Abdelrahman et al. (2012). Vayallil (2002) found that the antioxidant and antimutagenic activity in date fruit is quite potent, which suggests the presence of compounds with free-radical scavenging activity.

Perveen et al. (2012) observed varying degrees of growth inhibition in Fusarium, Aspergillus, Alternaria, and Trichoderma species, when exposed to extracts of date palm spathes. Aamir et al. (2013) tested the extracts and fractions for antimicrobial activity, and noted synergistic activity against standard microbial strains of *Klebsiella pneumoniae* (Gram-negative), *Staphylococcus aureus* (Gram positive), *E. coli* (Gram negative), *Salmonella typhi* (Gram negative), *Enterococcus faecalis* (Gram positive), *Pseudomonas aeruginosa* (Gram negative), and *Salmonella paratyphi* (Gram negative). *P. dactylifera* was observed to have a hepatoprotective effect in thioacetamide-induced hepatic necrosis in rats (Okwuosa et al., 2014).

Al-Taher's (2008) studies on rats indicate anticonvulsant properties of date palm spathes. Studies have also shown that constituents of dates have potent antioxidant, antitumour, and anti-inflammatory effects. Ajwah is the most medicinal cultivar. Studies attribute its anticancer properties to its high magnesium level. Ajwah dates are a natural source of folic acid, which helps mitigate cardiovascular diseases.

SYCAMORE

Though less well known than the common fig tree *Ficus carica*, whose fruit is renowned worldwide, sycamore was a sacred tree in ancient Egypt. *F. sycomorus* has a stately shape. Its leaves are smaller than those of *F. carica*, and resemble the leaves of the mulberry tree. The ripening of the fruit is hastened by manually incising the fruit a few days before harvesting. The white juice from the fruit and leaves is called the milk of the sycamore.

Sycamore remains date back to the third millennium BC in ancient Egypt. They are still found in the Egyptian delta region, and around oases. This long-lived tree can survive extended exposure to sun and drought, and was often planted alongside roads. The oldest sycamore tree in Egypt is in Matarria, a suburb of Cairo. The species also grows throughout Africa (south of the Sahara Desert), Southern Arabia, Lebanon, and neighbouring regions.

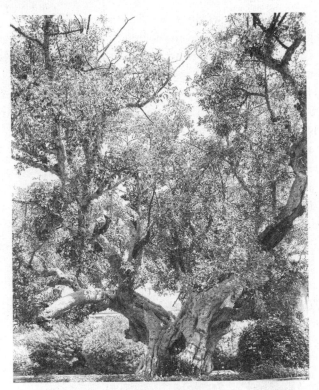

Figure 46 Old Sycamore tree from Israel, "Sycomoros old"
by Eitan f 14:23, 31 May 2006

Like the common fig, the fruit of this species can also be dried and preserved. The fleshy fruit of the tree is called the poor person's fig, because it is less sweet than the common fig. The leaves are estimated to have 9 percent crude protein, making it a preferred species as fodder for livestock.

The species helps fix sand dunes and improves soil, as falling leaves build soil humus and retain moisture. The softwood is pliable but easily damaged by termites and pests. The fruit can be fermented to make an alcoholic beverage, and leaves are used in soups, and other dishes. The latex in the sap is used to coagulate milk. The inner part of the root is used as weaving fibre, and a strong rope can be made from the inner bark. The bark is chewed with kola nut. In Ghana, the wood ash is commonly used as a salt substitute.

The bark is a dye source for traditional *bogolan* textiles in Mali and Burkina Faso in Africa. Bogolan comes from the African words *bogo* (earth) and *lan* (coming from). Bogolan textiles are dyed with mud that is rich in iron ore. The dye has a red-ochre to brownish color. These textiles are then hand painted with herbal dyes. Traditionally, tribal women dyed this cloth for festive occasions.

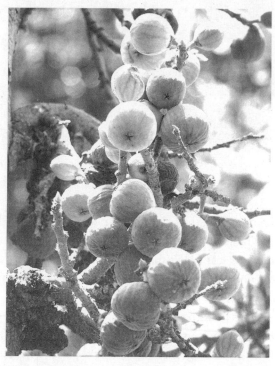

Figure 47 "Sycamore fruits" by Eitan f 13:46, 8 July 2006 (UTC), own work

In the dry desert regions of Egypt, the sycamore offered life-giving water, and it is referred to as the Tree of Life. Its fruit, timber, and twigs are represented in Egyptian tombs of the Early, Middle, and Late Kingdoms. The tree was thought to provide nourishment to departed souls in the afterlife. According to legend, two sycamores stood at the gateway of Heaven, and the sun god Ra emerged each morning from between these trees. Sycamores were regarded as manifestations of the Egyptian goddesses Nut, Isis, and Hathor.

By the reign of King Menkaure (c. 2739–2722 BC), Hathor, goddess of healing powers, was referred to as the Mistress of the Sycamore. Tomb paintings show Hathor leaning down from the tree to pour wine and offer bread to souls in the afterlife. The sycamore fig fruit was thought to possess intoxicating properties. The milk was used to heal wounds and abscesses, and the leaves were used to make funerary amulets. Coffins were made from sycamore wood, based on the belief that the dead person was in the womb of the mother tree goddess.

The Old Testament refers to the sycamore seven times and the New Testament, once. The number of references in the Old Testament underscores the ancient cultural connection between ancient Egyptians and Jews. The Talmud tractate Berkhoth mentions sycamore in reference to tithing. This tree was often placed near, or inside the necropolises. The wood of the tree was used to make coffins, water wells, and agricultural tools. Pliny noted that the wood can resist long periods of immersion in water.

The importance of fruit and timber trees like sycamore and cedar to the life of the people of the region is evidenced by numerous Bible verses like 2 Chronicles 9:27. In Luke 19:3–4, Zaccheus climbed a sycamore to see Jesus in the crowd. Rabbinical commentary on the Book of Genesis characterises the common or sycamore fig as the biblical tree of knowledge of good and evil. According to legend, Adam and Eve ate sycamore fruit in Eden, where the tree grew in abundance along the rivers.

The location of Eden is disputed, although it is widely believed that it lay between the Tigris and Euphrates Rivers, in current Iraq. A branch of sycamore was used to cover the nude bodies of Adam and Eve. It is also known as the Virgin Mary tree, because it is believed that the Virgin Mary took shelter under this tree. The Bible states that King David appointed an officer to look after the olives and sycamores (1 Chronicles 27:28). Psalms 78:47 refers to sycamore destroyed by frost.

Sycamore fruit and leaves were valued for their medicinal properties in ancient Egypt. The Hearst papyrus describes its calming effects and its use in treating hippopotamus bites. The milky latex was used to remove hair from the body, and the seeds were used to set bones and as a treatment for nails. The leaves treated snakebites and jaundice; the latex was found effective against chest diseases, cold, dysentery, ringworm, dysentery, and other skin diseases; the bark was used to treat respiratory ailments and scrofula; and the roots were found to have laxative, and anthelminthic properties.

With its antibacterial properties, the species also treats gingivitis. *F. sycomorus* proved to be more effective than insulin (standard treatment) at lowering blood glucose levels, in a dose-dependent manner in alloxan-induced diabetic mice (Njagi et al., 2012). *F. sycomorus* stem bark possesses a sedative effect, and has shown anticonvulsive properties in rats (Sandabe et al., 2003) The leaves demonstrate a wide range of insecticidal and ascaricidal properties, indicating that the plant could be developed as an organic alternative to synthetic pesticides (Romeh, 2013).

OLIVE

The olive tree is an evergreen, with dense, dark green foliage on the upper surface, and silvery gray leaves underneath. Olive flowers are white, small, and mildly fragrant. The tree rarely grows taller than 10 metres. The knotty trunk has many protuberances and coppices. The coppice shoots can be separated from the root to raise new plants. Olive trees can live for thousands of years. Pollen and fossil studies indicate that wild olives in the Anatolia region (modern Turkey) date back at least 50,000 years.

Fossilised olive trees from 50,000–60,000 years ago have also been found in the volcanic rocks of Santorini in Greece. From these, and other archaeological finds, it is likely that wild olive trees grew in the Aegean, Mesopotamian, and Biblical lands of Syria, Lebanon, Israel, and Turkey. The tree starts bears fruit when it is seven to eight years of age, and continues to bear fruit throughout its life. Crete has some of the oldest olive trees, including one that still bears fruit, and is estimated to be 3,000 years old.

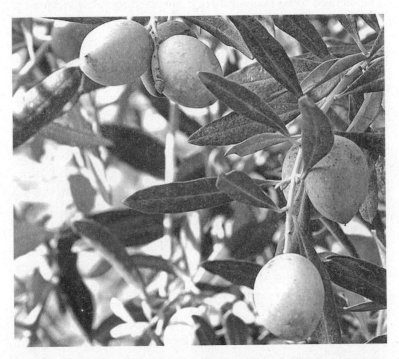

Figure 48 "Olives from Jordan" by Nickfraser

Olive cultivation perhaps began about 8,000 years ago at the end of the Neolithic period, in the Aegean region and in Syria. It was often done after consulting the stars, based on the belief that good harvests, and the position of the stars, are linked. Olives were then gathered by beating the tree with rods, and hand harvesting.

Pliny the Elder decried this practice in his *Naturalis Historia*: "Do not shake and beat your trees. Gathering by hand each year ensures a good harvest." Oil was extracted from the ripened fruits in stone and wood presses that were set up across the Mediterranean.

These have since been replaced by mechanical presses, though some traditional presses still exist in parts of the Mediterranean. The oil used to be pressed three times: the first press yielded the best oil, which is golden in color and lightly fragrant. Nowadays, oil extraction is done using centrifuges. The centrifugal process helps separate oil from the water and solids. This process can be passed through two or three phases, with each phase removing residual oil from the olives. The extraction processes also help remove a bitter substance known as oleorubin. The byproduct from oil extraction processes are used in soap making.

Nowadays, grafting of high-yielding cultivars on rootstock is common practice. The unripe fruit is green and turns black on maturity. An olive contains 10–40 percent oil by weight, and unripe and overripe fruits contain less oil. The oil contains palmitic, oleic, linoleic, stearic, and myristic acids and glycerides.

There are three categories of olive oils, based on acidity. Extra virgin olive oil is the highest-quality and has less than 1 gram of oleic acid per 100 grams of oil. This oil is often used for salad dressings and other foods. Virgin olive oil has more than 2 grams of oleic acid per 100 grams. Ordinary olive oil has more than 3.3 grams of oleic acid. Olives are preserved in salt solution, and used as condiments.

Olive trees and olive oil have played a pivotal role in the Mediterranean economy from the earliest of times. Ancient stone olive presses have been uncovered in Crete. Olive oil stored in large containers called *pithois* have been recovered from the Palace of Knossos (c. 1900 BC) in Crete. The Minoans who ruled Crete were the earliest people to cultivate the olive tree. Around 3500 BC, the knowledge of cultivation and hand harvesting of olive trees spread across the region.

An olive plant is often planted on the birth of a child, and again, as the child crosses various stages of life, from childhood to maturity. This tradition of tree planting has similarities with other religious traditions, like the Hindu tradition where tree planting has a strong association, and religious sanction. Olive wood is very hard and has a beautiful grain, making it valuable in ornamental furniture and fixtures.

More recently, the 2014–15 global production of vegetable oils is estimated at 176.95 million metric tonnes, of which olive oil accounts for just over 3 million metric tonnes. Most production (90 percent) is in the Mediterranean, with Spain accounting for 45 percent (3.2 million metric tonnes), followed by Italy and Greece.

Palm, soybean, sunflower, and canola continue to be oils that are more popular. With increasing focus on its health benefits, however, demand for olive oil is rising. More than 800,000 metric tonnes of olive oil is exported from the Mediterranean, according to World Olive Council data. In addition to Europe, Australia, and the Americas, Asian countries like India and China have shown increasing interest in olive oil.

Ancient Egyptians used olive oil in cooking, medicine, and in lamps. The Egyptians believed that the knowledge to produce olive oil was a gift from Isis, the goddess of agriculture. The desert regions of Egypt are at the edge of the olive tree range, so olives were likely imported into Egypt from Greece, Syria, and Palestine.

The oldest olive remains found in Egypt are charred stones from the Thirteenth Dynasty at Memphis (c. 1802–1640 BC).

Olive oil has been found in the remains of the ancient Egyptian worker villages, El Amarna and Deirel Medina, and olive trees have been found at Heliopolis (near Cairo). Recoveries from the Uluburun shipwreck off the southern coast of Turkey included Canaanite jars of olive stones, indicating that thriving olive trade existed from the southern coast of Turkey to Canaan and Egypt. Ramses III tried to cultivate olive trees in Egypt, but failed.

Olive imports must have put a substantial strain on the exchequer, and Ramses III was forced to use castor oil instead, in lighting, ointment, and perfume. Scented olive oil was used to perfume mummies, and stored in small alabaster and glass containers, which have been discovered in the ancient tombs of Egypt. The Tutankhamen tomb contains olive branches, and other flowers. Cleopatra used it as a skin softener in perfumed baths.

In Greek mythology, the olive tree is associated with fertility, strength, and victory. Homer called it liquid gold. According to myth, Zeus' daughter Athena struck her spear into the earth, and an olive tree grew there. Her namesake city, Athens, is said to be located on that spot. Hercules is said to have killed the Cithaeron lion with the help of an olive wood stake. Winners of the Olympic Games were crowned with a wreath of wild olive, and received a prize of olive oil. Athletes and gladiators applied olive oil on their bodies at games.

According to literature, the Athenian Games awarded the best runner 70 amphoras (each amphora contained 35–40 kilos of oil). Double this quantity was given to the chariot race winner. Spartans also anointed their bodies with oil prior to training. Olives were the main source of fat, as the Greeks regarded animal fat to be unhealthy, associating it with the barbarians. Olive oil was a sacred and offered to gods. It was processed by first blanching olives in hot water, stone pressing them, and then decanting the oil, and storing it in clay tubs.

The ancient Romans credited the goddess Minerva with the creation of the olive tree. During the initial years of the Roman Empire, Rome relied mainly on olives imported from its dominions of Greece, Spain, and other regions. Rome's conquest of Greece helped expand the cultivation of olive trees and olive oil production into new territories. Cultivation began in Italy, and eventually became a major source of revenue for the country. A vibrant trade in olive and olive products flourished in Roman territories. In war, it was common for defeated armies to carry olive branches to indicate surrender; today, the expression "extending an olive branch" means a desire for peace. Victors were honoured with olives.

Roman Caesars were crowned with wreaths of gold and olive leaves, and anointed with olive oil, similar to the ancient Biblical tradition of anointing Kings. With the fall of the Empire, olive cultivation in Europe declined for a millennium, but continued in Turkey and neighbouring areas. Production revived in the Middle Ages, and the olive was introduced in South America and North America, with the expansion of European colonies in the New World.

The olive appears on the seal of the United States of America: with the thirteen leaves and thirteen olives in the seal representing the Anglo Saxon people of the United States, who are thought to have descended from the thirteenth tribe of Ephraim of ancient Israel.

The olive tree, which was regarded as a symbol of love and peace, became an essential part of solemn rites, such as baptism. These practices were already part of the Hebrew tradition. The Olive tree in Hebrew is *es shemen*, which means "tree of oil." Thus, the practice of using olive oil in Orthodox churches is an extension of Hebrew, not Roman, tradition. The Bible contains twenty-five references to the olive tree and 160 references to olive oil. A bird carrying a twig of olive to Noah signaled the end of the flood.

Olive oil is the base of the Holy Anointing oil. Olive trees and oil were symbols of sovereignty used to anoint kings to the throne (1 Sam 10:1; 1 Kings 1:39). When David crowned as King of Israel, he was anointed with olive oil (Psalm 89:20). Thus, kings were called the "anointed ones." Isaiah 45:1 references Cyrus as God's anointed one. This practice has endured over millennia in Israel, and its neighbouring lands.

The culinary use of olives is also as ancient as the plant. They were regarded as the food of gods (II Chron 2:10). Given the olive's economic importance, there was a concerted effort to encourage its cultivation. Olive trees were planted across most of Northern African and the Mediterranean. Deuteronomy (8:8) states: "A land of wheat and barley, of vines and fig trees and pomegranates, a land of olive oil and honey."

There are at least seven references to the olive tree and olive oil in the Quran. Allah is the Light of the heavens and the earth. "The metaphor of His Light is that of a niche, in which is a lamp, the lamp inside a glass, the glass like a brilliant star, lit from *a blessed tree, an olive*, neither of the east nor of the west, *its oil all but giving off light* even if no fire touches it. Light upon Light. Allah guides to His Light whoever He wills and Allah makes metaphors for mankind and Allah has knowledge of all things" (Qur'an, 24:35).

The use of the oil is sanctioned in Islamic literature and writings. The famous Islamic scholar Ibn Al Qayyim, or Muhammad Al Bakr (1290–1350 AD), states that the red-colored oil is better than the blackish one. The red color is caused by pigment carotenoid and the blackish color from late-season olives. The oil continues to be prized by Palestinian Arabs, who mix bread, oil, spices, and salt for breakfast.

Olive oil has a wide range of medicinal properties. It is said that massaging the body with the oil helps heal hemorrhoids, ulcers, anal fissures, intestinal inflammations, and gastrointestinal tract ailments. It allegedly cures seventy diseases, including leprosy, pleurisy, cold, cough, and tuberculosis. Hippocrates mentions sixty conditions that could be treated with olives, including skin conditions, dental ailments, and gynecological ailments. It is regarded as an exhilarant that treats baldness, boils, digestion, and intestinal parasites. When mixed with common salt, it remedies oral diseases. Olive oil was used treat wounds, according to Isaiah (1:6).

Herbalists commonly use the olive leaf for its antiviral property. It is believed to lower blood pressure and to treat severe fever and tropical diseases, such as malaria. Crushed olive leaves were believed to be effective on boils, rashes, itching, and other skin diseases. Today, olive leaf extract is available from natural health practitioners and taken orally in tablet form.

Olive oil is a key ingredient in many skin healthcare products because of its ability to moisturise and nourish dry skin, strengthen weak and brittle nails, and restore luster to the hair and scalp. Hydration with a warm compress of the oil imparts a healthy look to skin. Fatty acids and phenolic compounds such as tocopherols help prevent skin damage, and have an antioxidant effect. This has led to extensive use of the oil in the pharmaceutical and cosmetic industry. Olive oil is popular carrier oil, and blends well with essential oils.

Modern scientific research has validated many traditional uses of olive. The American and British pharmacopoeias mention it. Numerous studies have indicated that the oil, rich in monounsaturated fatty acids, can be used by hypertensive patients. Several studies have validated that olive oil consumption helps prevent heart attacks, and other cardiovascular ailments. Fatty acids in the oil seem to decrease cholesterol levels, and have an anti-inflammatory effect.

In a study by the New York University Langone Medical Center, 232 people in the age range of twenty-five to sixty years, with high blood pressure, were randomised to receive olive leave extract (500 mg, twice daily), or a commonly used antihypertensive medication called captopril (12.5 mg, twice daily) for eight weeks. Both treatment groups experienced similar reduction in blood pressure levels.

Animal studies also weakly suggest that olive leaf might help control blood sugar levels in diabetes, and reduce symptoms of gout. Oxford University's Institute of Health found that olive oil may protect against colorectal cancer (Stoneham et al., 2000).

POMEGRANATE

Punica granatum, or pomegranate, is a small tree. The fruit contains acids, sugars, vitamins, polysaccharides, polyphenols, and minerals. Phenols (flavonoids and tannins) have been isolated from the pericarp, leaf, and flower. Complex polysaccharides have been detected in the peel. The seeds contain triacylglycerols with high levels of punicic acid. Seeds contain lignin, sterols, steroids, and cerebroside in very small amounts.

As the health benefits of pomegranates have become better known, the demand for pomegranates has increased, particularly in the United States. India accounts for 35 percent (900,000 metric tonnes) of the global pomegranate production. It exports fresh fruit to Dubai, where it is re-exported to Eastern Asia. Iran produces around 800,000 metric tonnes of fresh fruit annually, but exports a relatively small quantity (12,000 metric tonnes; 2007 estimate).

Iran also produces about 35,000 metric tonnes of pomegranate juice, which is rich in ascorbic acid, sugars, and tannins. Of this, 25,000 metric tonnes is exported to Europe, Canada, and the United States, mostly as concentrated juice.. Spain supplies fresh pomegranate to Europe, which absorbs 95 percent of its estimated production of 80,000 metric tonnes. Central Asia and

Afghanistan are new exporters of pomegranates. Afghanistan and neighbouring areas are famous for producing the best pomegranates.

The seed, which is a byproduct of fruit juice processing, yields pomegranate oil, which is rich in punicic acid. In some Iranian varieties, the total dry lipid content ranges from 66 to 193 grams per kilogram. The tannin in the skin of the pomegranate fruit is used to tan leather in parts of Africa. The main coloring agent in the pomegranate peel is granatonine. A solvent extraction method is used to extract the dye, which is used to dye cotton cloth.

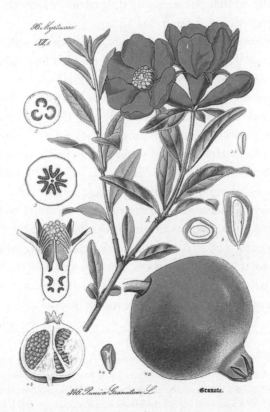

Figure 49 "Illustration Punica granatum2"

Most scholars agree that pomegranate originated from Persia. Archaeological discoveries from the eighth century BC indicate that pomegranate was an important fruit during the time of the Assyrians and Phoenicians. A vase decorated with pomegranates was discovered in a residence in Uruk (modern Iraq), which was founded by King Enmerkar (c. 4500 BC), and was the home of King Gilgamesh. Mesopotamian cuneiform tablets from the mid-third millennium BC mention pomegranates. Archeological evidence of pomegranate use was uncovered in Jericho in the West Bank and Ugarit, a port in Northern Syria. Settar and Korisettar (2001) indicate that pomegranate distribution extended from the Persian countries into the Indus Valley.

As previously mentioned, extensive trade existed between these regions. Thus, pomegranate likely traveled across the Biblical lands through trade. Persian mythology contains many references to pomegranate. Pomegranate represents fruitfulness, knowledge, learning, and wisdom. It is also a symbol of fertility and rebirth in ancient Persia and Greece. Isfandiyar, the famous Persian warrior, is said to have achieved immortality after eating a pomegranate fruit. Zoroastrianism, the monotheistic religion established in Persia, uses pomegranate fruit in marriage ceremonies.[2]

Herodotus mentions Persian warriors adorning their spears with golden pomegranates in the Persian War with the Greeks in the fifth century BC. In ancient Rome, brides wore headdresses made from pomegranate twigs. The ancient Greeks regarded pomegranate as a gift from Zeus, and believed that Persephone, the queen of the underworld, and goddess of crops, tied herself to the god of the underworld, Hades, by eating a few pomegranate

---

[2] Some scholars believe Aryans and Zoroastrians share common origins, as both originated in Central Asia along the borders of the Lake Baikal. Zoroastrians settled in Persia, and Aryans moved across the Hindu Kush Mountains and into the Indo-Gangetic Plains.

seeds. The dead were commemorated with an offering of boiled wheat and sugar, decorated with pomegranate. Today, Greeks break a pomegranate on the ground to initiate weddings, New Year's, and other celebrations, and pomegranate is often the first gift brought to a new home.

Ancient Egyptians buried their dead with pomegranates for use in the afterlife. Inscriptions depicting pomegranates have been discovered in burial sites of Tutmosi I (1547 BC) and Ramses IV (1145 BC). A silver vessel shaped like a pomegranate has been recovered from Tutankhamen's tomb in Egypt. Pomegranates are a fertility symbol in weddings among Bedouins. According to legend, each pomegranate seed comes from paradise and couples who eat fruit with abundant seeds will have many children. Bedouins also believe that pomegranates possess power over evil; thus, sleeping under the tree guarantees safety during the night.

In China too, pomegranates have similar symbolism. A pomegranate filled with seeds symbolises fertility. A picture of a half-open fruit is often given as a wedding gift. The seed in Chinese is called zi, which literally means "sons." A hundred seeds in a fruit thus symbolises a hundred sons. Traditional Chinese medicine prescribes pomegranate to treat infertility in women, as well as cough, indigestion, and other ailments. The Chinese pharmacopoeia mentions pomegranate.

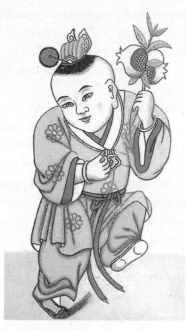

Figure 50 Pomegranate regarded as a fertility symbol in China,
"*Pomegranate China*" by Philg88], own work

Pomegranate is one of the seven staple foods consumed by the ancient Jewish people. It was believed that those who ate the fruit after thanking God for the goodness of the land would receive unique blessings. According to Jewish religious literature, the fruit has 613 seeds, equal to the 613 commandments of the Torah, illustrating its importance to the Hebrew people. It is Jewish tradition to eat pomegranate during Rosh Hashanah.

Some Jewish scholars regard it as the forbidden fruit of the Garden of Eden. Pomegranate appears as a holy symbol on ancient coins of Judea, and it symbolises righteousness. A pair of decorative silver pomegranates adorn the place where Torah scrolls are kept. King Solomon used the pomegranate fruit in the design of his crown. The Bible refers to the sacred pomegranate of Exodus, the secular pomegranate of Deuteronomy, and the sensuous fruit of Solomon's Song. The Quranic verses Surah 6:99 and 6:141 refer to grapes, olives, and pomegranates, as valuable fruit trees.

All parts of the fruit and plant are useful from a medicinal viewpoint. A decoction made from the seed is used to treat syphilis, and the juice is used to treat jaundice, diarrhea, nosebleeds, sore throats, coughs, urinary infections, digestive disorders, skin disorders, and arthritis. The fruit pulp and the seed are stomachic. Dried, pulverised flower buds relieve bronchitis. In Ayurvedic medicine, pomegranate is an antiparasitic, blood tonic, and remedy for aphthae, diarrhea, and ulcers. In Unani, pomegranate is a remedy for diabetes (Julie, 2008).

Dioscorides stated, "All sorts of pommegranats are of a pleasant taste and good for ye stomach . . . The juice of the kernells prest out, being sod and mixed with Hony, are good for the ulcers that are in ye mouth and in ye Genitalls and in the seate, as also for the Pterygia in digitis and for the Nomae and ye excrescencies in ulcers, and for ye paines of ye eares, and for the griefs in ye nosthrills . . . The decoction of ye flowers is a collution of moist flagging gummes and of loose teeth . . . ye rinde having a binding faculty . . . but ye decoction of ye roots doth expell and kill the Latas tineas ventris." Several early Roman medical writers recommended the use of pomegranate rind and root bark as a treatment for tapeworm infestation (*latas tineas ventris*).

The sterols, steroids, cerebroside, lignin, and derivatives in pomegranates were observed to possess remarkable antioxidant activities (Lansky and Newman, 2007). Studies indicate pomegranates could be useful in treating cancer, osteoarthritis, and other diseases. Studies also show that pomegranate seeds might help rid the digestive system of fats, a property that could have its application in weight loss therapy.

Clinical research indicates that pomegranates, when part of a healthy diet, might help prevent heart disease, heart attacks, and strokes. Pomegranates have the potential to thin blood, increase blood flow to the heart, lower blood pressure, reduce plaque in the arteries, and bring down bad cholesterol levels while increasing good cholesterol. Julie (2008) revealed that pomegranate juice could be used as a therapy in prostate cancer, particularly recurrent types. Other studies appear to validate these findings.

The juice helps in hyperlipidemia, because it decreases absorption and increases fecal excretion of cholesterol by affecting the enzymes that aid cholesterol metabolism. Pomegranate juice is also reported to be effective in reducing hypertension by decreasing angiotensin-converting enzyme activity, reducing myocardial ischemia, and improving myocardial perfusion.

Pomegranate juice could help treat diabetes and atherogenesis, through reduced oxidative stress. Other studies indicate a role of the fruit in treating periodontal disease and denture stomatitis. Other benefits may include combating bacterial infections, erectile dysfunction, male infertility, Alzheimer's disease, and obesity.

Pomegranate extracts are used extensively in skin care products especially due to their anti-inflammatory properties. They also extend the life of fibroblasts, the cells responsible for producing collagen and elastin that build, strengthen, and support the skin. As collagen fibres break down, skin ages and wrinkles. Pomegranate oil stimulates collagen production and increases flexibility in the epidermis and dermis, thus slowing the formation of wrinkles.

Studies have shown that pomegranate seed oil helps ameliorate some forms of skin cancer, perhaps because of its antioxidant properties. The oil helps control hyperpigmentation, and enhances topical effectiveness of sunscreen products.

WILLOW

The most likely botanical source of the willow mentioned in the Bible could be one of 400 species (e.g., *Salix alba*, *Salix acmophylla*, *Salix fragilis*, *Salix safsaf*, *Populus euphratica*). These species tend to grow in wet ground and along waterways, making them an excellent soil binder along riverbanks. Given the wide geographical dispersion and numerous species of willows in these lands, pinpointing a single species may not be possible.

Literature sources indicate that a small, willow-like tree was used to make furniture, tent poles, canes, and baskets. Funerary flints, shaped like willow leaves, date back to the Stone Age. A fishing net made from willow dates back to 8300 BC. Literature describes the trees as a source of pollen for bees.

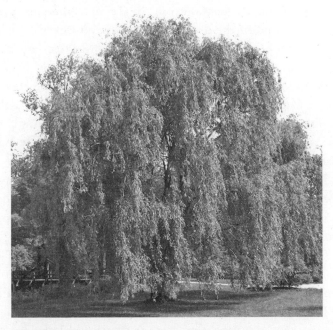

Figure 51 "Salix alba Morton" by Bruce Marlin, own work

Although not as revered as sycamore willow was prominent in ancient Egypt, and a primordial tree on which the sun rested in the shape of the benu bird. The willow tree was said to shade Osiris, god of the underworld, and protect coffins. Willow garlands have been discovered with the mummy Amenhotep I in the tomb of Tutankhamen.

Pliny mentions that a willow tree grew outside the cave in Crete where Zeus was born. The goddess Europa is pictured on Cretan coins sitting under a willow tree, and holding a wicker basket. Jehovah is worshipped on the Great Day of the Feast of Tabernacles, also called the Day of Willows. Belili, the mother of Sumer goddess Ishtar, was known as the Willow Mother. Samson was bound with shoots from willows (Judges 16:7).

The Scriptures contain six references to willow, and it is one of four species mentioned in the Talmud (the citron fruit, the closed frond of the date palm, boughs and·leaves of myrtle, and branches of willow). Branches of these four trees are waved during seven days of the annual Jewish pilgrimage festival Sukkot, commemorating the pilgrimage to the Temple. This practice has endured since the destruction of the ancient Temple of Jerusalem. The nostalgia of the willow is evident in Ezekiel 17:4–6 and other Bible verses. When the Jews, led by Moses, migrated from Egypt to Israel, they found willows near water.

The earliest references to willow's medicinal properties date from the third dynasty of the Kings of Ur in the Euphrates region of modern Iraq. This Sumerian civilisation, which flourished around 3000 BC, used willow as an analgesic, and anti-inflammatory. The Ebers papyrus and Hearst Medicine papyrus mention willow. The seeds of willow were recommended in the setting of broken bones, and the leaves were used to reduce wound inflammation. The Ebers papyrus mentions it as a salve ingredient for treating ear infections, and restoring suppleness to muscles and tendons. The bark and leaves were used to provide relief from painful arthritis.

Hippocrates and Dioscorides recommended willow bark for gout and rheumatic pain. Other ancient medicinal systems (Chinese, Assyrian, Greek, native North American, and Ayurveda) use willow for its analgesic, fever-reducing, and anti-inflammatory properties.

Today, the molecule acetylsalicylic acid, originally discovered in willow, is best known as aspirin. Studies conducted by New York University Langone Medical Center have explored using white willow as an alternative to aspirin, which is known to irritate or damage the stomach.

This side effect is significantly reduced in willow, perhaps because the active molecule salicin in willow is converted to acetyl salicylic acid (the irritation-causing molecule) only after it is absorbed in the body. Willow also contains less salicin than aspirin. Other molecules in willow could also depress the negative impact of active salicin. Double blind, placebo-controlled trials have found the plant to be effective for back pain, osteoarthritis, bursitis, dysmenorrhea, headaches, rheumatoid arthritis, and tendonitis.

MYRTLE

Myrtus communis is a small tree or shrub that grows from 10 to 24 feet and belongs to the guava and eucalyptus family. It is described as the queen of all sweet-smelling bushes in the world with shiny, dark green and scented leaves. The plant has white showy flowers and purple berries, which are dried before they ripen, so that they can be eaten. It prefers a mild subtropical climate, and cannot tolerate freezing conditions or dry winds. The species has disappeared from the Mount of Olives, but it grows in Samaria and Galilee (now Central Palestine). The species is believed to originate from the Mediterranean and Middle East, although others place it in Afghanistan and Iran.

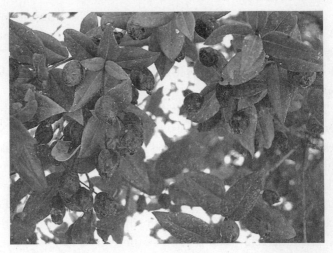

Figure 52 "Blue myrtle berries sardinia" by Japs 88, own work

Myrtle oil is extracted from leaves through steam distillation and its colour is clear yellow to greenish yellow. It has a camphorous and peppery smell, and is used in aromatherapy, cosmetic creams, lotions, and perfumes.

The principal constituents of the oil are camphene, cineol, geranial, linalool, pentene, myrtenol, and tannin. The leaves contain flavonoids such as quercetin, catechin, myricetin derivatives, and volatile oils, in addition to organic citric and malic acids.

The oil blends well with other essential oils like rosemary, benzoin, bergamot, eucalyptus, black pepper, cedar, frankincense, myrrh, neroli, rose, jasmine, lavender, lemon, lemongrass, coriander, ylang ylang, and sage. There are two varieties of myrtle essential oil. Green myrtle oil has a camphorous pine scent with notes of lavender, bay leaf, and eucalyptus. The red variety has a woody, peppery scent. The scents of both the varieties provide a top note that lasts for about 30 minutes.

In ancient Egypt, myrtle symbolised eternal life of the soul. The flowers represented the fleeting beauty of incarnate existence, because they quickly die and give way to bitter, dark blue berries. On the other hand, the evergreen leaves retain their scent.

In Greek mythology, myrtle is sacred to Aphrodite, the goddess of love, and Demeter, the goddess of harvest. Aphrodite (also known as Myrtila) was ashamed at her nudity, and hid behind a myrtle bush. In gratitude, she took the plant under her protection, and it became her favourite. Ancient Greeks and Romans planted myrtle around temples. It was believed to bring good luck. Soldiers, athletes, and nobles were honoured with a wreath of myrtle leaves. Women bathed wearing crowns of myrtle branches. Myrtle was used in wedding rituals. Farmers regarded the garland of myrtle as auspicious.

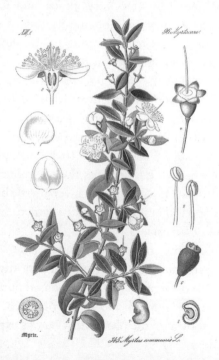

Figure 53 *Myrtus communis*, "Illustration Myrtus communis"

In *Tibb ul Nabi* (*Medicine of the Prophet*), the Prophet is purported to have said, "If anyone offers you myrtle as a present, do not refuse it. It is from the Heaven." In Islamic tradition, as in Christian and Jewish traditions, it is said that when Noah descended from the Ark, the first thing that he planted was myrtle. Myrtle was used to perfume water to wash the deceased. People visiting graves decorated them with myrtle twigs. In Turkey and Palestine, it was common to plant myrtle in Muslim graveyards.

Myrtle is a sacred tree for the Hebrew people. Nehemiah 8:15 states that myrtles grew on the hills around Jerusalem. The Talmud (Cuk 34; Yer Cuk 3, 53rd) describes the thick branches of trees as myrtle boughs. Jews regard myrtle as a symbol of sweetness, justice, divine generosity, recovery, peace, and God's promise. According to Sephardic tradition myrtle leaves were added to the water in the last (seventh) rinsing of the dead. During the Jewish festival of Sukkot, people wave branches of myrtle, citron, date palm, and willow. According to tradition, the myrtle branch used during Sukkot should have three leaves that emerge from a stem. Jewish women wore garlands of myrtle on their heads on their wedding day, as a symbol of conjugal love. Today, myrtle is carried with orange blossoms as a traditional bridal flower. In Jewish mysticism, myrtle represents the masculine force at work in the universe. The bridegroom was given myrtle branches before entering the nuptial chamber. Jews still use myrtle as a decoration at the Feast of Tabernacles.

Myrtle blossoms represent beauty, love, paradise, and immortality. According to Christian tradition, myrtle was given as a sacred plant to Virgin Mary. It symbolised purity and fertility. Myrtle is both the symbol and scent of Eden. According to legend, Adam took a myrtle plant when he was expelled from the Garden of Eden.

Food was often cooked on fires of myrtle leaf. Meat was wrapped with leaves steeped in wine and vinegar before cooking.

The edible berries were dried and used as a cheaper alternative to pepper, which was imported from India, and extremely expensive in ancient times. The dried, ground berry, called *mursins* in the Middle East, adds flavour to stews, jellies, and beverages. The roots and bark can be used to tan leather, giving it a distinctive aroma. It can also dye wool fibre for use in carpet weaving. Dried leaves boiled in water impart a mustard yellow color, which can be used to color yarns.

Nearly all ancient civilisations used myrtle to treat a range of diseases. Medicines were prepared by steeping the plant in wine and olive oil, and applying it as a paste. Ancient Egyptians knew of its antipyretic and anti-inflammatory properties. Dioscorides recommended wine in which myrtle leaves had been macerated, to treat pulmonary and bladder infections.

Islamic tradition involves a syrup made with myrtle to treat cough and diarrhea. An ointment made from leaves of sesame and myrtle was applied to sprains and burns. It was also said to relieve dysentery, eye disease, headache, urinary system ailments, and hemorrhoids.

In ancient Greece and rural Italy, myrtle berries were nibbled as a breath freshener. Myrtle has been traditionally used in Iran to treat malaria, abnormal uterine bleeding, and facial warts (Qaraty et al., 2014). In Ayurveda, it is used to treat epilepsy. Myrtle was also used to treat bronchitis infections and uro-genital problems in the nineteenth century (Annis Remedy, 2012; Begum et al., 2012). Women rubbed the leaves on their bodies to increase libido. A beverage infusion made of myrtle leaves was believed to enhance youth and beauty.

Myrtle leaves and flowers were used to make a popular skin care lotion called Angels Water in the sixteenth-century. They were also used to scent soaps, and toiletries. The oil is an insect repellent, thus myrtle branches were kept in kitchens. The oil is also effective in killing salmonella on fruits and vegetables. Washing with 1:1000 parts of myrtle leaf oil and water significantly reduces bacteria, and could thus be an alternative to chlorine and other synthetic disinfectants. The oil is also effective against *Candida albicans,* and many species of Aspergillus.

Recent studies have revealed that salicin is the active ingredient in myrtle. Amphotericin, an antifungal compound, has been isolated from the plant. A pharmacological review by Alipour et al. (2014) indicates that myrtle may possess antioxidant, anticancer, hepatoprotective, neuroprotective, and antidiabetic properties.

Myrtle could be a promising natural antioxidant, antigenotoxic, antimutagenic, and chemopreventive agent (Mimica-Dukić et al., 2010). Results from a study in Turkey appear to validate these properties (Serce et al., 2010). The antihyperlipidemic and antidiabetic properties have also been studied, with promising results (Alipour et al., 2014). In a comparison study using an antibiogram test, *M. communis* extract was found to be more effective than gentamicin against *K. pneumoniae, E. coli,* and *Pseudomonas aeruginosa* (Ahmed et al., 2013).

Studies have shown that myrtle oil reduces the size, secretions, and pain of mouth ulcers. Myrtoplex cream with 10-percent extract *M. communis* leaves is used to treat herpes simplex types 1 and 2. The main ingredients of this cream are tannins, polyphenols, and volatile oils, such as cineole and flavonoids. Panahi et al. (2014) found that the plant improved hemorrhoids.

Studies also show that the plants possess antiplasmodial (antimalarial) properties (Naghibi et al., 2013). Myrtle oil suppressed parasitic activity in mice (Dell Agli et al., 2012). It can also help stop hemorrhaging and minimise wrinkles by inducing the blood vessels to contract.

Myrtle is an astringent and a decongestant. Its adaptogenic properties help improve the health of thyroid glands, and have shown positive action in cases of hypothyroidism and hyperthyroidism. Trials on rats indicate reduction of blood sugar levels, a property that could be relevant to the discovery of new antidiabetic drugs. Studies have revealed that myrtle oil is a nontoxic, and effective mosquito repellent, similar to eucalyptus.

CHAPTER 5

CULINARY HERBS IN THE BIBLE

～∽～

Herbs and spices have played a critical role in improving the culinary experience of man over the millennia. This chapter focuses on culinary spices that were popular in Biblical times, when people relied on plants and trees for shelter, food, medicine, and spirituality.

ANCIENT CUISINE

According to the McCormick Science Institute papers, the most significant role of herbs was in healing, followed by food. Numerous references to the high cost of imported spices, especially those from outside the Mediterranean region, appear in Greek, Roman, Egyptian, Mesopotamian, Arabic, and Indian works. As described in Chapter 1, the vibrant spice trade in the first millennium BC and several centuries thereafter was controlled by the Phoenicians, who brought spices from the Land of Punt and India and charged high prices for them.

Ancient Egyptian Food

Although Egypt was the crossroads of the ancient Spice Route and had several Red Sea ports, the herbs and spices imported from the Land of Punt, the Islands of Malacca (modern Indonesia), and India would have been too expensive for most people. Only the rich could afford cinnamon, pepper, myrrh, and frankincense to season and enhance banquets of fowl and meat. Paintings of these grand banquets have been discovered at many prominent Egyptian archaeological sites. Thus, the cuisine of most ancient Egyptians was fairly simple.

Herodotus describes it as follows: "They eat loaves of bread of coarse grain which they call *cyllestis.* They make their beverage from barley, for they have no vines in their country. They eat fish raw, sun-dried or preserved in salt brine" (*Histories,* 2, 77). Many Egyptians relied on vegetarian food and what the Nile River and its flood plains provided. The most common seasoning was salt, along with locally produced herbs and spices like cumin, coriander, marjoram, dill, vinegar, and lettuce seeds. Mustard was cultivated in Egypt, probably starting in the Middle Kingdom (c. 2000–1700 BC). Coriander was prized as an aphrodisiac and its seeds, which symbolised eternal love and faithfulness, were planted in tombs as early as 1000 BC.

Ancient Greek and Roman Food

Romans and Greeks shared culinary customs, though each retained a unique identity. Greece and Rome both imported ginger from India and used cardamom as perfume. Both regarded garlic and leeks as aphrodisiacs. Anise-tasting fennel was popular too: the Greeks thought it made a man strong; the Romans thought it improved eyesight.

The Romans imported Indonesian cloves and nutmeg, which they regarded to be appetite stimulants. Romans used parsley as a garnish, but Greeks considered parsley to be sacred and not eaten. The Romans were particularly fond of rich sauces flavoured with vinegar, honey, and pepper, and herbs like dill, coriander, fennel, mint, oregano, cumin, saffron, myrtle berries, celery, sesame, anise, oregano, and lavender.

The history of Greek cuisine can be traced back 3,000 years. It is the forerunner of Western cuisine and spread via Rome, to Europe and beyond. The ancient Greeks prided themselves on simple, frugal food. Greece has a long coastline, so naturally its cuisine relies heavily on fish and other seafood. Vegetarianism was common, with food largely composed of wheat, olive oil, and wine. Meat was rarely eaten, although fish was more common.

Greek herbs included oregano, mint, garlic, onion, dill, bay laurel, basil, thyme, and fennel seeds. Cinnamon and cloves were also used in stews. The Persians introduced Greece to yoghurt, rice, sweets, nuts, honey, and sesame seeds. The conquest of Greece by Rome in 197 BC led to the introduction of sauces and pasta in Greek cuisine. Roman food is also rich in vegetables, low in meat, and influenced by cultural interactions with other nations.

Ancient Roman cuisine was perhaps the most interesting of the ancient cuisines. In early Rome, culinary differences between social classes was small. As Rome conquered more lands (e.g., Greece, Egypt, Assyria, Persia, Europe) and became wealthier, its cuisine also evolved. Expensive spices were imported for banquets through the port of Alexandria from around 200 BC. Pepper, which was extremely expensive and regarded as a symbol of wealth, was used in nearly every major recipe of ancient Rome.

In the first century AD, the satirist Persius wrote: "The greedy Merchants, led by lucre, run. To the parch'd Indies and the rising Sun; From thence hot Pepper, and rich Drugs they bear, Bart'ring for Spices their Italian Ware: . . ." Spice factories in ancient Rome manufactured combinations of popular spices. Liquamen, for example, was a sauce made from rotting fish guts, vinegar, oil, and pepper. It was regarded as an aphrodisiac. Among the recipes discovered at Pompeii were mushrooms with honey-and-liquamen sauce, soft-boiled eggs with pine kernels and liquamen sauce, and venison with caraway seeds, honey, and liquamen sauce. Another popular plant was laserpithium, the chief export from Libya and a primary spoil of the Punic Wars. It was roasted as a vegetable and the juice from the stems was used as flavouring. Within two centuries, laserpithium was consumed to extinction.

Descriptions of these ancient cuisines were recorded in several books and texts. Archestratos wrote the first cookbook in 320 BC, and Mithaceus was a cook and writer in the fifth century BC. Lynceus of Samos, a comedian around the fourth or third century BC, described Greek food in his writings. Hippolochus (c. third century BC) and Timachidas (c. 100 BC) also wrote about food. Additionally, several authors wrote about the eating habits of ancient Romans.

In 160 BC, Cato the Elder wrote *De Agricultura*, a treatise on agriculture with sections on cuisine. Columella's *De Re Rustica* is another famous work on agriculture written around the first century AD that contains about 500 recipes. Marcus Apicius, a gourmet and hedonist, compiled a comprehensive treatise on Roman food of his time.

Gaius Petronius Arbiter, a courtier who lived during the reign of Nero in the first century AD, refers to a lavish banquet called the Dinner of Trimalchio in his satirical novel *Satyricon*. Exotic food, opulence, and excess were the defining features of Roman banquets. Martial's *Epigrams* 1897 describes popular menus and food, especially during the *Saturnalia*, the most popular feast of the year.

Ancient Jewish Food

Ancient Jewish food was influenced by Egypt, Mesopotamia, Judea, Greece, and Rome, as well as Persian and Islamic traditions. High costs limited the use of herbs to local species (e.g., capers, coriander, cumin, black cumin, dill, dwarf chicory, hyssop, marjoram, mint, black mustard, saffron, and thyme) and a few imported spices (e.g., myrrh, galbanum, saffron, and cinnamon). Garlic and onions, and possibly fenugreek were eaten as vegetables, and used to season cooked foods. For special feasts, spices like pepper and ginger were imported by the wealthy and royalty from Arabia and India.

CULINARY HERBS

This section focuses on culinary spices that were popular in Biblical times: hyssop, wormwood, rue, coriander, cumin, dill, mustard, and mint.

Hyssop

The botanical source of hyssop, as with other Biblical plants, is shrouded in debate. The Bible mentions hyssop many times (Leviticus 14:1–7). A brush made of hyssop branches was used to mark houses of the Jews with lamb's blood to protect them from impending plague. David mentions hyssop in Psalm 51:7: "Cleanse me with hyssop, and I will be clean; wash me, and I will be whiter than snow." There are references to hyssop in the burning of the heifer (Numbers 19:6) and for sprinkling on a dead person (Numbers 19:18). In 1 Kings 4:33, Solomon "treated about trees from the cedar that is in Libanus [Lebanon], unto the hyssop that cometh out of the wall."

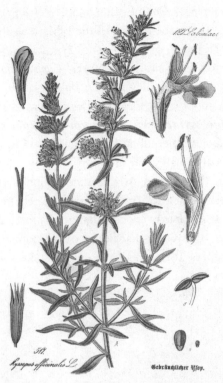

Figure 54 *Hyssopus officinalis*

Rabbi Saada Gaon (882–942 AD) and Maimonides (1155–1204 AD) believed that *Marjarano syriaca syn origanum syriacumsyn origanum maru* is the true hyssop, because it is identical to the Israeli *za'atar*. In Arabic, *za'atar* refers to marjoram and other genera in its family with similar scent and taste (e.g., thyme, satureja, savory) that are often used as marjoram substitutes. It is also called *ezov* in Hebrew and Biblical hyssop in English. Fleischer et al. (1988) concluded that Biblical hyssop was not *Hyssopus officinalis*, or *azob* in Greek, which means "holy herb."

Dioscorides wrote that hyssop was used to clean temples, similar to the Biblical descriptions of its use in Leviticus 14:1–7,

33–53 and Psalm 51:7. On the other hand, the *Encyclopedia Britannica* (2015) states, "Ezov, the hyssop of the Bible, a wall-growing plant used in ritual cleansing of lepers, is not *Hyssopus officinalis* . . . it may have been a species of caper or savory." *Capparis spinosa* is a caper found in the region. Stanley (2001), Balfour (1897), and several other authors support the idea that hyssop was *C. spinosa*.

Marjarano syriaca syn origanum syriacum syn origanum maru. *M. syriaca* is a perennial shrub that grows to a height of 30 to 60 cm. It bears small white and purple flowers. *M. syriaca* grows extensively in the eastern Mediterranean, including Israel, and from Northern Africa to Turkey, though rarely in the Egyptian Sinai region. It is a hardy species that grows in fallow, degraded, and rocky sites. Despite its hardiness, over exploitation has led to declining numbers. It is a legally protected species in Israel.

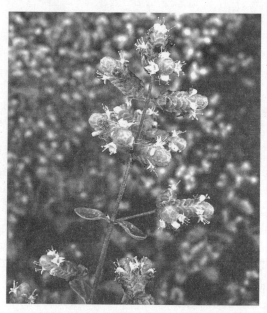

Figure 55 "Origanum marjorana 002" by H. Zell, own work

The leaves are used in the Middle East and Europe as a cooking spice in salad dressings, vegetables, and oils. Its aroma is similar to oregano, thyme, sage, and rosemary. The flavour comes out best when it is added at the end of the cooking process. The aromatic seeds are used in baked goods, sweets, and drinks, and fresh or dried leaves are used in herbal tea.

The famous culinary spice oregano also belongs to the genus Marjarano. Crowfoot and Baldensperger (1932) point out that the Samaritans have used this herb in the Passover ritual for more than 2,000 years. Furthermore, it is often observed growing out of rock masonry walls in Palestine, and it grows in the vicinity of Jesus' crucifixion site. According to the Bible, a branch dipped with vinegar was raised to the lips of Jesus on the cross. After receiving it, he said, "It is finished" (John 19:30). He then bowed his head and died. Such a branch would need to be long enough to reach Jesus' head, raised about one metre above the ground, thus ruling out *M. syriaca*. Yet, religious scholars argue that the cross may have been short, allowing a shorter branch to reach.

Traditionally, the plant is regarded as an antiseptic stimulant with antispasmodic properties. It is a good general tonic and is used to treat a variety of digestive and respiratory disorders. It is not recommended for use by pregnant women, as it can stimulate menstruation, though it is regarded as safe to consume in small quantities in food.

Chewing the leaves is said to help alleviate toothache. The species is used to treat muscular pain, arthritis, stiff joints, and sprains. The antioxidant properties of oregano have been studied and validated (Kizil et al., 2010). Dasgupta and Hammett-Stabler (2011) claim that *M. syriaca* can treat pain and respiratory ailments. Chieko et al. (2015) show positive results for the cytotoxic properties of the plant.

An essential oil is extracted from the leaves and flowers

by steam distillation and yields from 0.4 to 0.7 percent. Oil of marjoram is used in perfume, soaps, hair products, and food. Major volatiles and semi-volatiles isolated from the plant include α-pinene, β-myrecene, o-cymene, p-cymene, γ-terpinene, thymol, and carvacrol, many of which attract honeybees. The most active volatile ingredient, thymol, is used extensively for its antiseptic, antifungal, and antibacterial properties in over-the-counter mouthwash, cough syrups, and expectorants.

Hyssopus officinalis. *H. officinalis* is a perennial shrub that grows up to two feet. The stems have a woody base, and the plant bears white fragrant flowers. The plant grows in the wild in the Middle East, Southern Europe, and parts of central Asia. It is a naturalised species in the United Kingdom, and immigrants brought it to North America. The plant grows in rocky, dry, and stony locations, and in the cracks of old walls. It is a hardy species and can withstand desiccation. Beekeepers use the plant to attract bees and produce a pleasantly scented honey.

Harvesting is often done with flowers intact. The shoot is cut and dried in a cool, shady, and airy place to prevent discolouration. The spice, which has a sage and mint flavour, can be preserved for up to one and half years. Fresh and dried herbs and flowers are used as a spice in salads, soups, dessert, liqueurs, cakes, and other bakery products. It is widely used with wormwood, fennel, and anise to flavour absinthe. The leaves are used in Eau de Cologne and in liqueurs, such as Chartreuse. The spice is also used in perfumery, soaps, and cosmetics.

Medicinal properties of *H. officinalis* are also similar to *M. syriaca*. The herb is used in tonics for its calming effects. A poultice made from the herbs is used to heal wounds and reduce swelling caused by sprains. Tea made from the leaves is used to treat flatulence and stomachache. Hyssop is believed to irritate the mucous membranes, thus herbalists recommend its use only when the infection of the respiratory tract has subsided. The plant should not be used by pregnant women; when ingested in large quantities, it can induce miscarriage.

In the sixteenth and seventeenth centuries, a hot infusion with vapors was used to treat ear ailments. The bruised leaves were rubbed on rheumatic joints to relieve pain. The juice from the leaves was used as an insect repellent, and to remove lice and intestinal worms. Some people use hyssop as a gargle and bath oil (WebMD). The muscle-relaxing property has been indicated in trials on guinea pigs by Lu et al. (2002). The antimicrobial, antifungal, and antioxidant properties have been tested and validated in animal trials (Kizil et al., 2010). The U.S. FDA declared hyssop "Generally Recognized as Safe," although convulsions in rats have been observed during experimental trials.

Just like *M. syriaca*, an essential oil is extracted from the shoots by steam distillation. The oil is pale yellow to brownish yellow in colour, and average yield is about 0.6 percent. The oil is used in aromatherapy but only under expert supervision, as it can cause convulsions. According to Mitic et al. (2000), the main components of the oil are cis-pinocamphone (42.9 percent), trans-pinocamphone (14.1 percent), germacrene D-11-ol (5.7 percent), and elemol (5.6 percent).

The oil has a camphoraceous, herbaceous, spicy, earthy, and woodsy fragrance. It blends well with angelica, basil, bergamot, cajeput, camphor, celery, sage, clove, eucalyptus, fennel, geranium, lavender, lemon, lime, myrtle, orange, rosemary, and sage (www. ElizabethVanBuren.com). It is used to treat skin, digestive, and respiratory ailments. The oil may be used in a nebulizer diffuser, and in acupressure and reflexology.

Artemisia Absinthium (Wormwood)

This herbaceous perennial plant can grow to a height of two to four feet. It has silvery white leaves and stem, and a bitter taste. It is widely distributed in the Mediterranean, central Asia, Europe, and Kashmir. It is a native to temperate regions of Europe and a naturalised species in the United States. The plant is found in the wild and cultivated as an ornamental.

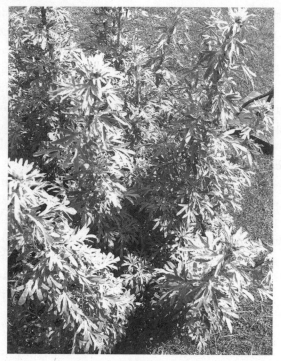

Figure 56 "Artemisia absinthium P1210748" licensed under CC BY-SA 3.0 via Wikimedia Commons

In Biblical times, wormwood was a symbol of calamity and sorrow: there are seven references to wormwood in the Old Testament, including Deuteronomy 29:18, Proverbs 5:4, and Jeremiah 9:15, and only one in the New Testament (Revelations 8:11). However, it had important medical uses. The Egyptians used wormwood as an antiseptic, stimulant, aromatic essence, tonic, beer and wine additive, and remedy for fevers and menstrual pains. The

Greeks, who called it *apsinthos,* had similar uses. They also used it in childbirth.

Hippocrates Corpus recommends wormwood to women suffering from menstrual pain and anaemia. The Romans referred to it as *absinthium,* roughly translated as "bitter." Wormwood was thought to counteract most of the poisonous effects of hemlock and toadstools. Roman soldiers would place the herb under their sore feet for relief. It was also used as an additive to rice wine in China (Ratsch, 1998, p. 70). The plant was used to expel intestinal worms in Egypt, Greece, and Rome, until the Middle Ages.

Today, Bedouin Africans sell wormwood in Egypt as a remedy for ill health. The Bedouin also burn wormwood leaves as incense around their newborn children. They believe that this will bring good health to the child. Traditionally, wormwood was ground into powder and burnt on coal fire or in incense smudge bundles. Dried wormwood herb was also smoked.

The plant is indicated to possess both neurotoxic and neuroprotective properties in studies conducted on rats (Lachenmeier, 2010). A 10-week study conducted in Germany evaluated the potential benefits of wormwood for treatment of people with Crohn's disease, an inflammatory condition of the intestines (New York University Langone Medical Centre, 2014). Most people who received wormwood showed gradual improvement of symptoms. Initial preliminary indications hint that wormwood essential oil (like many other essential oils) might have antifungal, antibacterial, and anti-parasitic actions.

Common wormwood is a relative of sweet wormwood (*Artemisia annua*), an ingredient in traditional Chinese malaria treatments, and in the pharmaceutical antimalarial drug artemisinin (also called artemesin). It is also used in an artemisinin-based combination malaria treatment. Combination malaria treatments, as opposed to single-drug treatments, reduce the risk of parasites developing resistance.

Wormwood essential oil is a dark green to bluish liquid of medium consistency with a spicy, warm, bitter-green odour and sharp, fresh top note. Wormwood contains the essential oil absinthol. It blends well with ambrette seed, jasmine, lavender, neroli, and oakmoss. The distilled oil is concentrated and must be used with care. It should not be used in aromatherapy. It has hallucinogenic properties and can cause nightmares, convulsions, vomiting, and even brain damage. Its active ingredient is thujone, which is chemically similar to tetrahydrocannibol, the active ingredient in marijuana. Thujone is a close organic cousin of menthol, and in its purest form, thujone has a minty aroma. Thujone is said to contribute to nerve depression, severe mental impairment, and eventual loss of reproductive function. Thujone can be found in cooking spices, such as sage, and other spirits like vermouth and bitters. The U.S. FDA has banned thujone in all foods and alcohol.

Wormwood (*Artemisia absinthium*) is the key ingredient of the controversial aperitif known as absinthe. It was also used in other wines and spirits, including bitters and vermouth. By the end of the nineteenth century, absinthe had acquired legendary fame among artists and Bohemians. Famous artists like Toulouse-Lautrec, van Gogh, Picasso, Gauguin, and Manet worked under the influence of absinthe. Van Gogh was severely addicted to absinthe. His work reflects the enhancement of colour and swirling alteration of reality, which is associated with its hallucinogenic effects. The following verse by Oscar Wilde exemplifies the thinking on absinthe in the artistic community of the time: "After the first glass you see things as you wish they were. After the second, you see things as they are not. Finally, you see things as they really are, and this is the most horrible thing in the world."

Ruta graveolens (Rue)

Ruta graveolens is the botanical name of rue. This perennial grows to an average height of about one metre and emits an offensive odour. It is native to the Mediterranean and India. The Spanish brought the plant to Latin America, where it dispersed widely in the tropical regions south of Mexico, and some temperate parts of North America.

As a culinary herb, rue was used sparingly in ancient Greece but extensively in ancient Rome. Today, rue and its oils are used sparingly in Italian and northern African cuisine as an aperitif in alcoholic beverages and an additive, particularly in Ethiopia. It goes well with acidic flavours and is added to pickles, capers, meats, cheeses, and eggs. In Latin America, rue is added to salad.

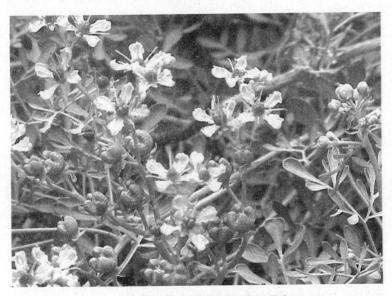

Figure 57 "Ruta graveolens3" by Kurt Stüber

Luke 11:42 enunciates the importance of this herb in the Palestinian region, as Jesus refers to a tithe on rue. Because the Bible describes the period from about a thousand years before the birth of Jesus, it is possible that rue grew wild then, with cultivation starting around the time Jesus was born. The Talmud describes rue as a kitchen herb that grows in the wild. Thus, it is not unexpected to exempt wild plants from tithing. Nevertheless, Christians regard rue as a cultivated species.

The Greeks also valued the herb. In his *Materia Medica,* the Greek physician Dioscorides states: "Boiled with vinegar it easeth pains, is good against the stitch of the side and chest, and shortness of breath upon a cold cause, and also against the pain in the joints and huckle bones . . . The juice of Rue made hot in the rind of a pomegranate and dropped into the ears, takes away the pain of thereof . . . That Rue put up in the nostrils stayeth bleeding." He also describes two kinds of rue: a mountain variety and a strong-smelling garden variety. The garden plant was tithed and apparently cultivated even then. Soranus, a gynaecologist in second-century Greece, described it as a potent abortifacient.

The Romans grew rue around their temples to Mars. It was regarded as sacred to Diana, the moon goddess, and Aradia, purported in legend as her daughter. Roman philosopher and healer Pliny mentions rue 80 times in his work. He states, "when notwithstanding it is of power rather to procure bleeding, through its sharp and biting quality. The leaves of Rue beaten and drunk with wine are an antidote against poisons, as Pliny saith." Pliny also reported that, in ancient Rome, painters and engravers used rue to sharpen and preserve their eyesight.

Rue was believed to provide protection against plague. People rubbed their floors with fresh rue to repel fleas and used it as an insect repellent for hundreds of years. According to legend, King Mithradates of Asia Minor survived his enemies' attempts to poison him by eating rue. The Turks kept pots of rue in their drawing rooms for its scent. Early Christians called it the Herb of Grace and used it during exorcisms and before Mass. During the Middle Ages, Christians sprinkled holy water containing a sprig of rue to protect against witchcraft and spells during Sunday mass. The native peoples of North America, Aztecs, and Mayans made extensive use of rue (Vogel, 1970, 78, 413).

Given the fairly widespread distribution of the species in the Mediterranean, the Arabian Peninsula, South America, and Africa, its use as a herbal remedy with many applications is not surprising. All ancient herbal medicine systems, including Ayurveda and Unani, use it for arthritis, gastric and respiratory ailments, and infections and ailments of the mouth. Rue leaves contain rutin, an antispasmodic flavonoid. Rutin has a beneficial effect on the circulatory system. It is recommended in herbal treatment of insomnia, headaches, nervousness, abdominal cramps, and renal trouble. Traditionally, it is regarded as a contraceptive and a well-known emmenagogue. The most frequent use of the plant has been to induce abortion.

The plant may be part of sedative and hypnotic herbal preparations. Like other bitters (e.g., wormwood), rue has been used as a dewormer. It was also used to treat pulmonary conditions such as tuberculosis, to reduce swellings of the spleen, and to treat wounds, varicose veins, and rheumatism. In European herbal medicine, the plant was often used to relieve hysteria, epilepsy, vertigo, colic, poisoning, and eye problems. Rue has been used to treat leukoderma, vitiligo, psoriasis, multiple sclerosis, cutaneous lymphomas, and rheumatic arthritis.

Since Pollio et al. (2008) discovered that rue can be fatal if ingested, its use as a medicinal and culinary herb has diminished. A significant temporary immobility of spermatozoa without any adverse effects on other sperm characteristics was observed in *R. graveolens L.* aqueous extract trials conducted on rats. Thus, the plant has potential use as a male contraceptive. The antioxidant potential of *R. graveolens* was investigated and validated in preliminary experiments.

Homeopathic trials indicated prospects of using the species as an anticancer drug (Freyer et al., 2014). Rue oil is a powerful local irritant (Martindale, 1982). Combined with other herbs in homoeopathy, it is used as an antiviral agent and rubefacient to treat eczema and psoriasis (Vigneau, 1985).

The analgesic property of the species has been studied by Nauman et al. (2012), who tested it against the standard allopathic drug diclofenac and attributed its effectiveness to flavonoids. Pandey et al. (2011) tested its effectiveness against a range of bacteria (e.g., *P. aureus, E. coli, P. aeruginosa, K. pneumonia, S. aureus, Bacillus subtilis, S. typhimurium, Aeromonas culicicola*) and fungi (e.g., *A. niger, A. flavus, Penicillium crysogenum, Rhizopus stolonifera*, and *Fusarium oxosporium*) and noted positive results.

Coriandrum sativum (Coriander)

Coriandrum sativum (coriander) belongs to the Apiaceae family. It rarely grows taller than half a metre. The flowers are arranged in umbels, and the small globular fruit produces the famous spice. The characteristic smell of the green plant is caused by aldehydic compounds (terpenes, linalool, and pinene). The leaves and seeds are rich in calcium, magnesium, manganese, iron, and vitamin C.

Its origin may be in Southern Asia and the Mediterranean, but it is cultivated around the world. *C. sativum* yields two crops per year: one in summer and one in winter, depending on day length and temperatures. Coriander produces a considerable quantity of nectar that attracts insects, bees, and moths. Luk'janov and Reznikov (1976) find that honeybees can produce up to 500 kg of honey from a hectare of coriander.

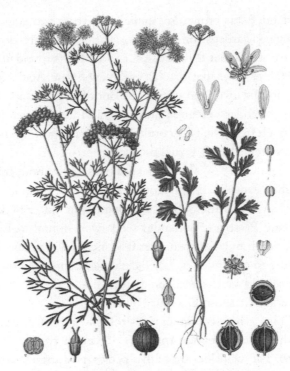

Figure 58 *Coriandrum sativum* by Franz Eugen Köhler

Current world production of coriander fruits is difficult to estimate, because official statistics as a separate crop are not available, and data from home and small gardens are not captured. Diederichsen and Axel (1996) estimate that the worldwide annual cultivation area of coriander is 550,000 hectares and annual production of coriander fruits is 600,000 tonnes. The main producers of coriander fruits are the Ukraine, Russia, India, Morocco, Argentina, Mexico, and Romania. The main exporters of coriander are the Ukraine, Russia, India, and Morocco. Main importers are the United States, Sri Lanka, and Japan, followed by Malaysia, Chile, Bolivia, and some countries in the Middle East.

Coriander was grown in Persia 3,000 years ago and scented the hanging gardens of Babylon. The oldest archaeological evidence of coriander may be the coriander fruits found in Israel's Nahal Hemel Cave that date to the New Stone Age (Neolithic era), before the invention of pottery. Both Egyptians and Greeks believed coriander was an aphrodisiac, and it was regarded as a symbol of eternal love. Dioscorides wrote that ingesting coriander could heighten a man's sexual potency.

Van Harten (1974) argues that the Jews knew about coriander before they came to Egypt around 2000 BC. Coriander, which grew in Egypt and the Sudan, was one of the bitter herbs used to celebrate Passover. Coriander seeds were found in Egyptian tombs (c. tenth and ninth centuries BC), including Tutankhamen's. References to coriander as a medicinal plant appear in the Ebers papyrus and in tablets recovered from the destroyed library of Ashurbanipal (c. seventh century BC).

In China, where coriander was probably imported via the Silk Route, the earliest mention appears to be in the fifth century AD (Li, 1969). The white blooms of the species have attracted mention in the Bible. In the Bible, the spice is compared to manna, a gum exudate that was a source of sustenance for the Jews during their exile from Egypt.

The plant is a popular spice in cuisines worldwide. The leaves and seeds are often ground into a powder and used as a condiment. In India, coriander has been in use perhaps as long as it has in Egypt. It is an essential spice in Indian homes used in curry powders, pickling spices, baked goods, meats, fish, and tobacco products.

In Ethiopia, coriander is used to add flavour to *berbere,* a spicy pepper blend used in meat and vegetarian dishes (Fossil, 1996, pers. comm.). Coriander also flavours alcoholic beverages like gin and is said to enhance the inebriating effect. The famous Russian rye bread *Borodinskij chleb* is spiced with coriander. In China, the roots are used in cuisine.

The essential oil content of ripe and dried fruits of coriander varies from 0.03 to 2.6 percent and fatty oil from 9.9 to 27.7 percent (Diederichsen, 1996). Both essential and fatty oils have industrial applications, though modern alternatives are preferred. The essential oil is extracted through steam distillation and used in food and cosmetics. Like the fruits, it is a carminative.

It is more stable and retains its scent longer than any other oil of its class. Decylaldehyde (yield 0.1 percent of the weight of coriander oil), obtained by treating the oil with bisulphite, is reported to be useful in perfumery (Diederichsen, 1996). The commercial oil is adulterated with sweet orange oil, cedar oil, turpentine, and anethole or aniseed oil (Bhatnagar, 1950). The main component, linalool, is used as a base for further technical processing.

Traditionally, coriander is used in the preparation of many household medicines to treat colds, fever, nausea, vomiting, indigestion, worms, rheumatism, epilepsy, anxiety, insomnia, and joint pain. In India, the fruits are used as a carminative, diuretic, tonic, and stomachic, as well as antibilious, refrigerant, and aphrodisiac. It is an external treatment for ulcers and rheumatism (Hegi, 1926).

Losch (1903) describes how the fruit must be soaked in wine or vinegar overnight before re-drying to remove chemical compounds that cause dizziness. Many of coriander's healing properties are attributed to phytonutrients and bioactive compounds (Rajeshwari et al., 2011). These include aliphatic lactones, terpenes, glycerides, anthraquinones, sterols, and essential oils. It can also reduce lipid levels, perhaps because of its ability to increase bile synthesis. The species has shown anti-arthritic, anti-inflammatory, antioxidant, antimicrobial, anxiolytic, anticonvulsive, antidepressant, and neuroprotective properties in animal trials.

Haggag (2011) found that nephrotoxicity and hepatotoxicity decreased in rats fed with *C. sativum*. It can conceal the taste or smell of other ingredients in pharmaceutical preparations (Jansen, 1981). The herb may help prevent oxidative stress-related diseases and enhance the effectiveness of conventional treatments (Tang et al., 2013). *C. sativum* does not appear to affect testosterone or cholesterol levels, or reproductive or endocrine functions (Al-Suhaimi, 2008). Human clinical trials to validate its hypoglycemic property have been successful.

The essential oil showed pronounced antibacterial and antifungal activity against Gram-positive (*S. aureus*, Bacillus spp.) and Gram-negative (*E. coli*, *S. typhi*, *K. pneumonia*, *P. mirabilis*) bacteria, and the pathogenic fungus *C. albicans* (Matasyoh et al., 2009). De Almedia et al. (2014) showed antifungal potential of *C. sativum* leaves. Khani et al. (2012) demonstrated biological activity of the essential oil against adults of *Tribolium confusum Duval* (confused flour beetle) and *Callosobruchus maculatus F* (cowpea seed beetle), indicating its potential as an insecticide for grain crops.

Cuminum cyminum (Cumin)

Cuminum cyminum, or cumin, is an annual herb of the parsley family. It rarely grows higher than one metre and bears flowers in umbels. It is native to India, the Mediterranean, Europe, Iran, and regions of Asia and Africa. It is an introduced species in Mexico, Latin America, and the United States.

Cumin oil is extracted by steam distillation from the ripe seed. It is pale yellow in colour and acquires a deeper yellow colour as it ages. The oil has an overpowering smell and blends well with caraway, angelica, rosemary, and chamomile. Although nontoxic, the oil is phototropic and exposure to the skin can cause dermatitis. The oil is useful in treating muscular aches.

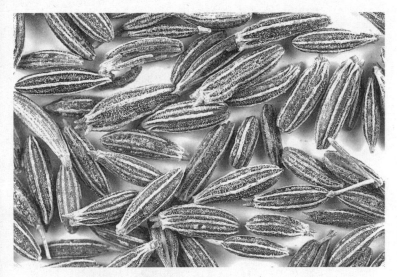

Figure 59 Cumin seeds, "Sa cumin" by Sanjay Acharya, own work

The spent cumin from which oil has been extracted contains 23 percent carbohydrates, 19 percent protein, 10 percent fat, and 5.5 percent soluble dietary fiber. It also contains thiamine (0.05 mg/100 g), riboflavin (0.28 mg/100 g), and niacin (2.7 mg/100 g). It is a rich source of minerals: Fe^{2+} (6.0 mg/100 g) and Zn^{2+} (6.5 mg/100 g). Monoterpene, hydrocarbons, oxygenated monoterpenes, oxygenated sesquiterpenoids, saturated and unsaturated fatty acids, aldehydes, phenolics, flavonoids, and tannins have been identified in the plant.

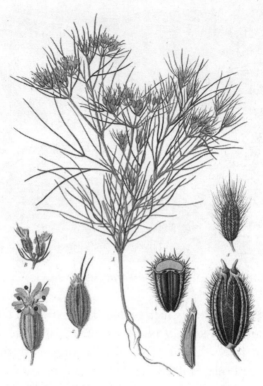

Figure 60 *Cuminum cyminum* by Franz Eugen Köhler

India is the largest producer, consumer, and exporter of cumin in the world. In 2009–2010 India's estimated production was 290,000 metric tonnes, domestic consumption was 100,000 metric tonnes, and global consumption was 187,000 metric tonnes (Indiabulls Commodities Limited). According to the government-operated Indian Spices Board, whose main objective is to expand and export spice production, India exported 49,750 metric tonnes of cumin in 2009–2010.

Other major producers of cumin are Syria (10,000–20,000 metric tonnes), Iran (5,000–10,000 metric tonnes), and China (8,000 metric tonnes). Some production takes place in Mexico,

Portugal, Spain, Japan, Netherlands, France, and Morocco. Syria and Turkey consume 10 percent of cumin; the rest is exported to Europe, the United States, and Latin America. With supply outstripping demand, the market price of cumin is low, thus future cultivation may be reduced.

Ancient Egypt, Greece, Rome, and China were producers and consumers of cumin. Cumin seeds have been recovered from multiple ancient Egyptian archaeological sites. Papyri from 1550 and excavated pottery from the fifth century BC include a cough remedy that has cumin, honey, and set milk as ingredients (Poole, 2001). The Pharisees collected tithes on cumin, indicating its importance to the local economy.

In one of the oldest ancient Egyptian medical texts, the Hearst papyrus (c. second half of the second millennium BC), cumin seeds are mentioned as medicine and as indigenous to Egypt. Various prescriptions are given in paragraphs 28, 55, and 125. "The seeds were considered to be a stimulant and effective against flatulence. They were often used together with coriander for flavouring. Cumin powder mixed with some wheat flour as a binder and a little water was applied to relieve the pain of any aching or arthritic joints. Powdered cumin mixed with grease or lard was inserted as an anal suppository to disperse heat from the anus and stop itching."

The spice was well known to ancient Greeks and Romans. Greeks kept cumin at the dining table, similar to pepper today, and this practice continues in Morocco. Cumin was regarded as a good substitute for black pepper, which was an expensive import from India. Pliny wrote that ground cumin seed in bread, water, or wine aided digestion and treated squeamishness, similar to the Egyptian practice.

Ancient Romans and Greeks used cumin in cosmetics to create a pale, pallid complexion. Pliny also suggested that smoking the seeds would give a desirable "scholarly pallor." Socrates considered it beneficial as an aid to scholarly pursuits. Cumin represented faithfulness, and soldiers and merchants sometimes carried the seeds in pockets, to remind them of family waiting for them back home. In ancient Rome, in addition to being a valued spice, cumin was regarded as a symbol of avarice and greed. Marcus Aurelius and Antoninus Pius, emperors with a reputation for their avarice, were privately nicknamed "Cuminus."

Verses written after the death of the Prophet Isaiah, who is said to have been born in the Kingdom of Judah (c. eighth century BC), indicate that cumin was an important spice in ancient Israel. With the rise of Islam in the seventh century AD and the Mongols in 1206, the trade routes and supply chain between the Middle East and Europe were severed. Jews emerged as the sole neutral traders. However, inter-regional trade was limited and the spice became less abundant in Europe during the Middle Ages. Eventually, Spanish and Portuguese colonialists introduced the spice to the Americas as European colonial powers gained control of these lands in the sixteenth and seventeenth centuries.

The primary medicinal properties of cumin are in the seeds, which are carminative, antispasmodic, antibacterial, astringent, antimicrobial, antidiabetic, anti-inflammatory, and analgesic. Cumin is an emmenagogue and galactogogue. It is used to relieve mild digestive disorders, diarrhoea, dyspepsia, morning sickness, colic, dyspeptic headache, and bloated stomach. The hepatoprotective property of the plant has also been indicated in animal trials. Cumin is a popular folk medicine in India to ease flatulence.

In the Middle East, a decoction of cumin seeds mixed with ginger, basil, and honey is a remedy for cough, cold, and flu. In India, black pepper is added to this mix. Mixing cumin with dried mint leaves helps clear bronchial and nasal passageways. In Arabia, cumin is mixed with black pepper and honey for use as an aphrodisiac.

In Ayurveda, a decoction of cumin seeds in water is given to stimulate the appetite and as a general nutritive tonic to improve heart health and cognitive function, and nourish the eyes. In Traditional Chinese Medicine, cumin is often integrated into medicated teas to treat cough and fever, or in food to aid digestion.

Whole, dried cumin seeds may be chewed as a remedy for nausea or dizziness and as a breath-freshener. Tisanes made from cumin have also been employed to soothe muscular spasms. In the past, it was used to treat epilepsy and tremors. A poultice or a plaster can be applied to bruises, swellings, stitches, and sore muscles to facilitate healing and prevent infection. Applied topically, it may help fight fungal diseases. It was once employed by ancient Indians and Egyptians as a remedy for headaches, and mental and physical exhaustion. When combined with spices like cinnamon and resinous gums like myrrh or frankincense, it was considered a potent and enervating aphrodisiac. It is believed that excessive use of cumin could be harmful to pregnant women and could even lead to miscarriage, nausea, and mild stomach upsets. Cumin has been used as a hair-rinse, and if first steeped in vinegar, it is said to help fight dandruff, to darken and thicken hair, and encourage hair growth. Whole crushed cumin seeds may be macerated in a base oil and applied as a general analgesic, rubefacient, and disinfectant. Spent cumin may be added to food to improve digestibility and nutrient composition (Milan et al., 2008).

The essential oil of cumin is derived from steam distillation. It can be mixed with natural waxes, esters, or base oils to create salves, balms, ointments, or liniments. In aromatherapy, cumin essential oil may relieve spasms, general muscular discomfort, anxiety, nausea, nervousness, and stress. Many of its traditionally regarded medicinal properties have been studied.

The potential use of cumin seed essential oil against *K. pneumonia* in vitro has been validated by Derakhshan et al. (2010).

The oil was also found to be a potent antimicrobial agent against *E. coli* strains by Bokaeian et al. (2014). Saboo et al. (2014) found that cumin was a potent antidiarrhoeal in rats. Jagtap et al. (2010) found that cumin has antidiabetic properties, and Dhandapani et al. (2002) claim that the spice is more effective than glibenclamide in treating diabetes mellitus.

The chemo-preventive potential of cumin seeds to modulate carcinogen metabolism has been studied (Gagandeep et al., 2003). Sayyah et al. (2002) found that administration of the essential oil at anticonvulsant doses can produce sedation and motor impairment in maximal electroshock, and pentylenetetrazole-induced tonic seizures.

Bunium bulbocastanum and *Nigella sativa* (Black Cumin, Black Seed, Fitches)

Black cumin, whose Biblical origins are unclear, is a popular spice across the globe. Reviews of papers and ancient literature suggest two candidates: *Bunium bulbocastanum* and *Nigella sativa*. *B. bulbocastanum* is the botanical name for black cumin. This species is native to Northern Africa and parts of Southern Europe.

It is a perennial herb that grows to a height of just over half a metre. The tubers are quite small. The roots and leaves can be eaten cooked or raw. When cooked, it has a sweet chestnut flavour. The seed and flowers of the plant are used as food flavour and as a substitute for cumin. The leaves are used as a garnish and flavouring, much like parsley.

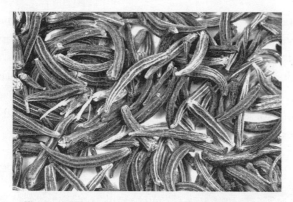

Figure 61 "Black Cumin" by Sanjay Acharya, own work

N. sativa ("black seed") is a species found in Southern Asia, the Arabian Peninsula, and Europe. It is an annual herb that grows to height of less than one foot. The herb bears white to light yellow delicate flowers. *N. sativa* seeds are used across India, the Middle East, and the Mediterranean region in cooking and in traditional medicine.

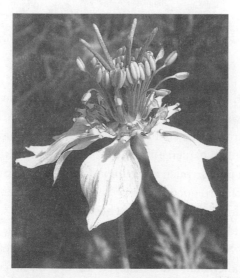

Figure 62 *Nigella sativa* in Vienna Botanical Garden by AndreHolz

In India, black cumin used in cuisine as well as in medicine. Moreover, *B. bulbocastanum* is restricted to the northern state of Kashmir and its availability across Southern Asia is subject to production and supply constraints. According to hadith, the Prophet Muhammad is believed to have said: "In the black seed is healing for every disease except death" (Sahih Bukhari). This indicates that the spice was available locally in Arabia.

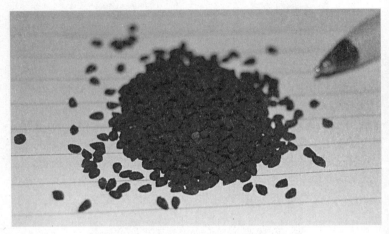

Figure 63 "Nigella seeds" by C94wjpn

Black cumin seeds have been known to the Egyptians, Assyrians, Greeks, Jews, Romans, Indians, and northern Africans since antiquity. Archaeologists found a bottle of black cumin oil in the tomb of Tutankhamen (c. 1350–1323 BC), which is currently displayed at the Egyptian museum in Cairo. Egyptian papyri show that physicians frequently prescribed the seeds after extravagant feasts to calm upset stomachs. They also used the seeds to treat headaches, toothaches, colds, and infections.

Queen Nefertiti (c. 1370–1330 BC), the chief spouse of Pharaoh Akhenaten, was believed to use black cumin oil to strengthen and bring luster to her hair and nails. Cleopatra (69–30

BC) is also stated to have used the oil for health and beauty. The Assyrians mention the use of black cumin seed to treat stomach ailments and skin conditions like itching, rashes, sores, and herpes. They used it externally on the eyes, ears, and mouth. It was used as a culinary spice too. The use and importance of black cumin, also called fitches in the ancient Mediterranean and Western Asia, is apparent from Isaiah 28:27 and Ezekiel 4:9 in the Bible.

Cumin was exported from Egypt to Imperial Rome, where it was used in medicine and food. The spicy seed was used to preserve meat and flavour food such as curries, pastries, and cheese. The Roman food writer Apicius wrote a recipe for a pear omelet that uses black cumin as spice. In India and Afghanistan, black cumin seeds are traditional toppings for flat breads. When roasted, the seeds add aromatic flavour to curries, biryani, pickles, and masalas.

In Northern Africa, the seeds are used in couscous and ground meat dishes. It is an ingredient of the popular spice blend called *Baharat* in the Arabian region. Throughout the Middle East, the spice is added to cakes, confections, alcoholic beverages, scents, and candies. Cooking oil is also produced from the seed. An infusion made from crushed seed steeped in boiled water is quite popular.

All herbal medicine systems (e.g., Unani, Tib, Ayurveda, Siddha[3]) regard the seeds and oil as useful in treating a range of ailments. In Unani, black cumin seed is mentioned as an important remedy. Hippocrates recommends black cumin, or *melanthion* in

---

[3] Siddha medicinal systems are among the earliest herbal medicine systems in Southern Asia. Siddha probably originated at the time of the Indus Valley civilisation in the second millennium BC before the advent of Ayurveda. The Aryans pushed it into the southern parts of India. Its herbal and medicinal practices are similar to those of Ayurveda, perhaps because of the close interaction between the immigrant Aryans and the indigenous Indian people. For more information about Siddha, see the upcoming book, Herbs from the East.

Greek, to treat digestive and liver ailments. Dioscorides used the spice to treat intestinal parasites, toothaches, headaches, respiratory congestion, and amenorrhea. He also used it as a diuretic and to enhance lactation. Pliny the Elder in his *Naturalis Historia* lists black cumin for snake bites, scorpion stings, old tumours, abscesses, and skin rashes. Egyptian seeds grown in near perfect-conditions around oases were especially prized.

In Arabo-Islamic culture, black cumin has been prescribed for various ailments including fever, asthma, chronic headaches, diabetes, digestion, back pain, infections, and rheumatism. In Arabic culture, black cumin is known as *Habbatul barakah*, the seed of blessing. In fact, since its rise in popularity in the seventh century, it is still regarded as an important family medicine and the oil that is most often used medicinally. Ibn Sina, also known as Avicenna (980–1037 AD), mentions it in his *Cannon of Medicine*: "that which stimulates the body's energy and helps recover from fatigue or dispiritedness." The spice is also believed to be good for purification and detoxification of the body; reduction of mucous and improved lung function; fever, coughs, and colds; toothache; headache; skin diseases and wound treatments; intestinal parasites and worms; and poisonous bites and stings.

The medicinal properties of the species have been tested in modern research. Khan et al. (2013) have found the plant to be effective against *S. aureus*, depending on the extraction solvent and processing methodology. The fruit extracts have been tested in studies of diabetic complications and aging (Ahmed et al., 2014).

According to the Memorial Sloan Kettering Cancer Center, various scientific studies indicate that molecules from the plant have immune-modulating, antioxidant, antiparasitic, and hepatoprotective properties, indicating that the seed of *N. sativa* may be useful in treating asthma, hypertension, rheumatoid arthritis, dyspepsia, diabetes, dermatitis, and even cancer. The

U.S. FDA have granted two patents for use of the oil to treat cancer-related ailments and improve immune systems.

Haq et al. (1999) demonstrated the immunomodulatory effect of proteins in *N. sativa* seeds through experiments. Dada et al. (1995) also found that the species had a hepatoprotective effect on rats. Other scientific studies show that the seed and oil are cardioprotective (El Tahir et al., 1993) and gastroprotective (El-Abhar et al., 2003). These studies give scientific rigor to the Prophet Muhammad's teaching that black cumin can treat every ailment. However, as is the case in most herbal medicines, further investigation must be conducted to corroborate these findings and support the development of new drugs.

Anethum graveolens (Dill)

Anethum graveolens (dill) can be a perennial or annual herb, depending on where it is cultivated. The plant normally grows to a height of under one metre. It was perhaps a native of the Mediterranean and central Asia. Its geographical distribution has since expanded, and the herb now grows around the globe.

Dill contains monoterpenes (limonene, carvone, and anethofuran), flavonoids (vicenin and kaempferol), vitamins, (A and C), minerals (folate, iron, and manganese), and amino acids. Oil yield is about 3.5 percent. Oil extracted from the leaves and seeds is used in beauty and skin care products. The oil is pale yellow in colour and darkens over time. Japan and India are major exporters of dill oil. The oil from India has a lower carvone content.

Dried dill foliage is commonly called dill weed and is used to flavour meats, sauces, stews, breads, vinegar, and pastries in Asia, Europe, and the Americas. It is a popular pickling spice in the United States. The aroma is sweet and tangy, between anise and caraway. Fresh herbs have a stronger fragrance than dried. The fragrance vanishes when overcooked, so it is best to add dill when food is nearly cooked.

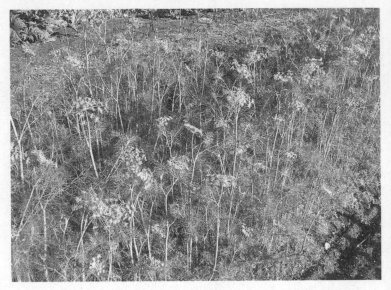

Figure 64 Dill plants in the field, "Anethum graveolens 001" by H. Zell

The name dill derives from the Norse word *dilla*, which means to soothe. It was regarded as a plant that helps allay pain. According to Zohary and Hopf (1988), the earliest evidence of dill cultivation is from a late-Neolithic lakeside settlement in Switzerland. Ancient Egyptians believed that dill possessed aphrodisiac and soothing properties, and they used it ward off evil. The Ebers papyrus mentions dill as an ingredient in a pain-relief mixture prepared by Egyptian physicians. Several twigs of dill were found in the tomb of Amenhotep II (1427–1401 BC).

Dill was extensively cultivated in Biblical lands from the time of Isaiah the Prophet (c. eighth century BC). The Bible contains multiple references to dill. Greeks and Romans burnt dill-scented oil as a sign of wealth. The Romans thought that dill had fortifying qualities, and gladiators ate dill for strength. The English regarded it as a magical herb and good-luck plant that repelled witches. Dill branches were hung outside doors in Europe to ward off evil.

Brides put dill in their shoes, along with a pinch of salt, for good luck. Charlemagne (eighth century) ordered dill bouquets placed on banquet tables to use as a digestive aid.

Dill was popular with ancient Greeks and Romans, who attributed to it a range of medicinal properties. Hippocrates advised the use of a liquid dill concoction as a mouthwash. Dioscorides recommended making a strong tea from the dried leaf and seeds to cure inhibited lactation, difficult urination, hiccups, flatulence, and uterine problems. He applied scorched dill to soldiers' wounds. Galen recommended dill weed as a sleep aid. Pliny the Elder mentions dill in his *Naturalis Historia*.

Herbal physicians still recommend dill to improve digestion, relieve hiccups, gas, diarrhoea, insomnia, arthritis, cold and cough, painful urination, kidney disorders, menstrual disorders, pain, and dysentery. They also recommend dill for oral care, bone health, and diabetes. Dill seed freshens breath and can alleviate throat and mouth pain. Dill weed sprigs are regarded to be antiseptic, digestive, and carminative.

The essential oil eugenol in dill has been used as a local anaesthetic and antiseptic. Eugenol also has been found to reduce blood sugar levels in diabetics. It may be used on the scalp to get rid of lice. Dill essential oil is also used to treat muscle cramps, intestinal spasms, and colic (it is an ingredient of gripe water).

Dill oil may be used in combination with chamomile to alleviate symptoms of attention deficit hyperactivity disorder in children. It acts as a mild sedative and has a calming effect on the brain. It is used to relieve anxiety, anger, and depression. It also helps to induce sleep at night. The U.S. FDA considers dill essential oil to be a food additive and has classified it as "Generally Recognized as Safe."

Pharmacological studies have validated some traditional medicinal properties of *A. graveolens*, including its antimicrobial, anti-inflammatory, analgesic, gastric mucosal protective, and antisecretory potential. It relaxes smooth muscles and increases progesterone. A powder of *A. graveolens* leaves significantly reduced lipids in hyperlipidemic patients (Sahib et al., 2012). Except for reduction of the atherosclerotic index, its effect is comparable to that of the standard agent lovastatin (Sahib et al., 2012).

Its ethyl acetate content provides antioxidant effects, which might explain its antihyperlipidemic and antihypercholesterolemic effects (Bahramikia et al., 2008). According to some studies by cosmetologists and dermatologists, dill may have anti-aging abilities because of its elastin protein, which helps maintain skin firmness.

Arora et al. (2009) found considerable antibacterial activity against a range of pathogenic bacteria. However, Sharopov et al. (2013) showed that the essential oil had limited effectiveness against *E. coli*. Singh et al. (2006) showed that dill essential oil may be a natural antimicrobial and antioxidant. The essential oil extracted from the seeds of *Anethum graveolens L.* was demonstrated in experiments by Jun Tian et al. (2012) to be an ecofriendly antifungal agent.

The antimycobacterial property of dill was demonstrated by Stavri et al. (2005). A 2006 study in the *Journal of Food Science* showed that dill essential oil was effective against several bacteria strains, inhibiting the growth of *Fusarium graminearum*, *S. aureus*, and other bacteria. Another study at the University of Vienna found that dill extracts from seeds stored for 35 years killed several fungal strains, such as *Aspergillus niger*, *Saccharomyces cerevisiae*, and *Candida albicans*.

Mustard

Mustard plants come from several plant species. The most common mustards are *Brassica alba* (yellow or white mustard), *Brassica juncea* (brown or Indian mustard), and *Brassica nigra* (Black Ingra or black mustard). All species are pungent, with the highest level of pungency found in black mustard and the least in white mustard.

The pungency comes from its isothiocyanate compounds, which develop after grinding the seed in cold water. Grinding releases the enzyme myrosin, which acts on a sinigrin glycoside molecule to produce a sulfur compound. Mustard oil is obtained from the seeds. This pungency decreases if the oil is boiled or mixed with other ingredients.

Greeks and Romans used mustard as a condiment and ground mustard seed with wine to make a meat sauce. The spicy seed was a popular condiment in the Han Dynasty in China (206 BC– 221 AD). European emperors in the sixteenth and seventeenth centuries regarded mustard as a valuable condiment.

Mustard was introduced to North America by Europeans and remains one of the most popular spices in that region today. *B. alba* (white mustard) is the mildest and is used to make traditional American yellow mustard. *B. juncea* (brown mustard) is dark yellow, has a pungent taste, and is used to make Dijon mustard. It is easier to harvest brown mustard seed than black mustard seed, which fell out of use in commercial products in the 1950s.

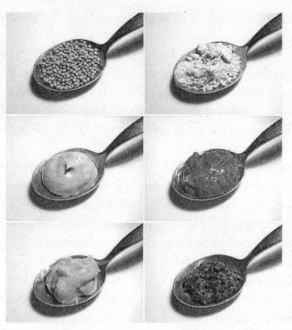

Figure 65 Mustard seeds (top left); ground mustard seeds (top right); table mustard with turmeric (centre left); Bavarian sweet mustard (centre right); Dijon mustard (lower left); French mustard from black mustard seeds (lower right)

B. alba is an annual species that probably originated from the Mediterranean, although it is now found across the world. A teaspoon of *B. alba* seed contains 87.1 mg of omega-3 fatty acids, 84.2 mg of omega-6 fatty acids, 22.2 mg of potassium, 27.3 mg of phosphorous, 9.7 mg of magnesium, and 16.9 mg of calcium. It is a popular condiment in many parts of the world, particularly Greece and Southern Asia.

All parts of the mustard plant and its oil are eaten in salads, curries, stews, and soups in Southern Asia. On the Indian subcontinent, a less pungent oil, called Newari oil, is produced from roasted mustard seeds. This oil has a deep brown colour and a smoky, full flavour not unlike Chinese sesame oil. The oil is used as a seasoning in various cold dishes in Nepali and Indian cuisine.

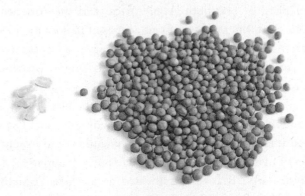

Figure 66 White mustard seeds compared with rice seeds, "Sinapis seeds" by Edal Anton Lefterov

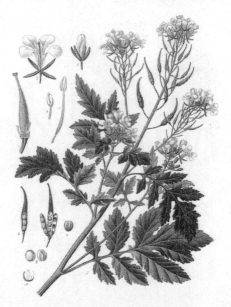

Figure 67 *Brassica alba* by Franz Eugen Köhler

B. juncea is the common brown mustard used in Europe, China, Southeastern Asia, and India. It grows as a weed in Southern Russia and Siberia, the Caucasus, and Central Asia, and as a casual or feral plant in Southern Asia, Africa, and the Americas. Oil extracted from the seed is refined and used in cooking in Russia and parts of Asia. This oilseed is also grown as a spice crop in North America, mainly in the Canadian prairie provinces of Manitoba, Saskatchewan, and Alberta.

B. nigra, or black mustard (named after the black seed) is used as a condiment and medicine in the Mediterranean region and India. In India, it is known locally as *rai* and is used in relish and pickling of mangoes, chilies, and other foods. It imparts a distinct flavour to curry. It is also cultivated as a vegetable in Northeastern Africa. *B. nigra* is an annual herbaceous plant that rarely grows beyond two metres in height. Mustard blooms are yellow and the fields of mustard when in bloom are a carpet of yellow.

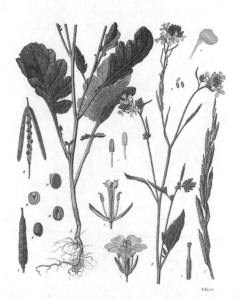

Figure 68 *Brassica nigra* by Franz Eugen Köhler

Canada produces 200,759 metric tonnes of mustard seed and has 57 percent (141,660 metric tonnes) of the global market share, followed by Nepal, Ukraine, and Myanmar. According to 2010 FAO estimates, Nepal produced 149,625, Ukraine 64,400, and Myanmar 58,300 metric tonnes of seed. If including the entire global production of mustard, then India produces an average of 6 million metric tonnes of rapeseed (mainly from *B. juncea* and *B. campestris*), which far exceeds Canada.

However, its high erucic acid content makes it unsuitable for global export, so most of this mustard is used locally in cooking oil, soaps, and earthen lamps to illuminate temples of Hindu gods (although this practice is disappearing with modernisation). Oilseed cattle feed, popular with cow farmers, is a byproduct of the oil extraction industry. FAO statistics show that the United States is the biggest importer of mustard seed, accounting for 24 percent (64,812 metric tonnes) of global imports, followed by Germany (17 percent) and Bangladesh (12 percent). American and European consumption is nearly exclusively in the form of condiments and spices, whereas in Bangladesh and other Asian countries it is mostly cooking oil.

Mustard is one of the oldest spices used by humans. According to an allegorical story by Gautama Buddha (c. 563–480 BC), the Buddha asked a grieving mother who lost her only son to bring a handful of mustard seeds from a family that has never lost a child, husband, parent, or friend. When the mother was unable to find such a family, she realised that death is common to all and thus she should not be selfish in her grief.

In the Quran too, God states that the scales of justice on the Day of Judgment will measure even a mustard seed's amount, because God is the most efficient reckoner. Jewish texts compare the knowable universe to the size of a mustard seed. An intimate connection between the small mustard seed and faith occurs in the Bible, Quranic Hadiths, and Hindu literature.

The relationship between mustard and faith is mentioned in the Gospel of Matthew and others. Mustard represents insignificance of the self and the world in the eyes of God. Mustard also represents humility.

Mustard seeds have been discovered in tombs of Pharaohs. They were thought to bring good luck. With the expansion of the Roman Empire, mustard traveled to Gaul, Spain, and England. King Charlemagne introduced mustard in the gardens surrounding the monasteries of Paris, establishing the now famous mustard industry in France. A 1634 law granted exclusive mustard-production rights to Dijon, now famous for its mustard. In German folklore, brides sewed mustard seeds into their dresses to bring them strength in their new home, perhaps because women were treated as subordinate to men and mustard brought good luck. In Northern Europe, mustard seed was said to keep evil spirits away.

Mustard seed is often used in herbal medicine. Hippocrates used mustard in many medicines and poultices. Pythagoras mentions mustard as a remedy for scorpion stings. Mustard was said to increase blood circulation. Mustard plaster helped increase blood flow to inflamed areas and thus hasten healing. By drawing the blood to the skin surface, mustard relieves headache, neuralgia, and spasms. Mustard was thought to be an aphrodisiac in Europe and China. When taken in sufficiently large doses, it warms the body.

Mustard was used to relieve toothache, muscle cramps, clogged sinuses, and indigestion. French monks used mustard to treat wounds. A rubefacient poultice provided relief of rheumatic pain. Hot water poured on bruised seeds makes a stimulating bath that is good for achy feet, colds, and headaches. Mustard has been used to treat alopecia, epilepsy, snakebite, and toothache. The seed is also used internally as a digestive, diuretic, emetic, and tonic. Mustard oil is said to stimulate hair growth, and it is a popular hair oil in rural India. However, direct application of the oil has been known to cause severe irritation.

B. alba is not used as medicine in developed regions of the modern world. In China, it is used to treat phlegmy cough, tuberculosis, and pleurisy. Limited human evidence supports the use of mustard plaster for bronchitis or mustard oil for preventing heart attack. Moreover, evidence is conflicting as to whether mustard oil is effective at lowering cholesterol. *B. alba* is traditionally used as a massage oil in Southern Asia. Its beneficial effect has not been scientifically examined.

B. juncea seed is a warming, stimulant herb with antibiotic effects. The medicinal properties of the species are similar to *B. nigra*. The seed is used in the treatment of tumours in China. The Chinese eat the leaves in soups to treat bladder ailments, inflammation, and hemorrhage. The root is used as a galactagogue in Africa. The odour repels mosquitoes.

In Java, the plant is used as an antisyphilitic emmenagogue. Leaves applied to the forehead are said to relieve headache. *B. juncea* has hepatoprotective properties that may be useful for treating liver disease (Gupta et al., 2011). The aqueous seed extract of *B. juncea* has shown potent hypoglycemic activity in male albino rats, indicating antidiabetic use of the seed (Tirumalai et al., 2011).

Jasim (2012) found that antibacterial action of *B. nigra* seed oil against Staphylococci and Escherichia species in the dental plaque of children one to five years old was comparable to that of gentamycin and ciprofloxacin. Stoin et al. (2007) showed the antibacterial property of *B. nigra* against multiple pathogenic bacteria.

Kiasalari et al.'s (2012) experiments on mice show that the *B. nigra* seed extract can be used in grand mal seizure treatment, probably because of its antioxidant property that acts via an enzyme activity mechanism. The pungency of the oil of *B. nigra* is from erucic acid and isothiocyanates, which are said to cause accumulation of triglycerides in the blood and thus considered bad for the heart; however, human trials have not been conducted to confirm these negative health effects.

Nevertheless, in the United States and parts of Europe, mustard oil is permitted for external use only and it cannot be sold as cooking oil. Canola oil from crossbred *B. juncea* seeds is permitted for use in food, because this oil has very low levels of erucic acid.

Mentha Genus (Mint)

Mint belongs to the Mentha genus and has dozens of species and cultivars. Hybridization between species occurs naturally. The four most commonly cultivated species are *Mentha arvensis* (Japanese mint, menthol); *Mentha piperita* (peppermint); *Mentha spicata* (spearmint); and *Mentha citrata* (bergamot). *Mentha sylvestris* is another wild mint that grows much larger than *M. spicata*. This species was used in the Middle East and Israel, as a condiment and in medicine. Scholars think that *M. sylvestris* is likely the mint mentioned in the Bible.

All are herbaceous plants, readily sending out runners and stolons. New roots and shoots emerge from nodes. The plant can be separated in between nodes and propagated. The name mint derives from Mintho, a beautiful nymph loved by Pluto, the Greek god of the underworld.

Aerial shoots and foliage are sources of essential oil rich in menthol, carvone, linalool, and linanyl acetate. Mint is rich in vitamins A and C. It also contains small amounts of vitamin B2 and the minerals calcium, zinc, copper, and magnesium. Spearmint oil is similar to peppermint oil but slightly sweeter and pale yellow to greenish in colour. Dried peppermint typically has 0.3–0.4 percent volatile oil containing menthol (7–48 percent), menthone (20–46 percent), menthyl acetate (3–10 percent), menthofuran (1–17 percent), and 1,8-cineol (3–6 percent).

Peppermint oil also contains small amounts of additional compounds including limonene, pulegone, caryophyllene, and pinene. The compound carvone gives spearmint its distinctive smell. Spearmint oil also contains significant amounts of limonene, dihydrocarvone, and 1, 8-cineol. Unlike peppermint oil, oil of spearmint contains minimal amounts of menthol and menthone. Oil is extracted by steam distilling the flowering tops of the plant.

M. piperita (peppermint) is a globally distributed hybrid of *Mentha aquatic* (watermint) and *M. spicata* (spearmint). Its name derives from its unique peppery flavour. Peppermint is a relatively new addition to the mint family and herbal medicine. It was first described in 1696 by English botanist John Ray (1628–1705), who discovered it growing in a field. It was admitted into the *London Pharmacopoeia* in 1721. The species has been extensively cultivated across North America since 1855, and the United States is now the most important producer of peppermint oil.

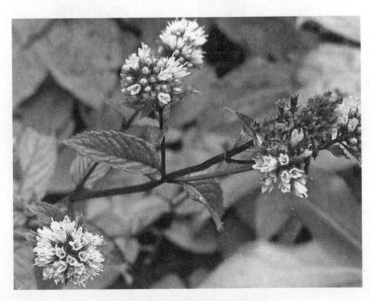

Figure 69 "Mentha-piperita" by Sten Porse

M. spicata grows well in nearly all temperates to subtropical climates. It grows to a height of two feet. It is native to the Mediterranean but is now globally distributed. The dark green, lance-shaped, jagged leaves have a sweet flavour with a cool after taste. The flowers are usually pink, pink-lilac, or sometimes green. Spearmint leaves can be used fresh, dried, or frozen and can be preserved in salt, sugar, alcohol, or oil. Harvesting is done at the onset of flowering or when flowering reaches its peak, after which leaves lose their aroma. The herb is cut about one-half to three-quarters way down the stalk (leaving room for smaller shoots to grow).

M. spicata has a milder flavour compared to peppermint. It is used in candy, gum, teas, meats, fish, curries, salads, beverages, vinegars, jellies, and sauces, as well as in toothpastes, cosmetics, and skin-care products. Spearmint dressings are particularly popular in summer in Greece and Southern Asia.

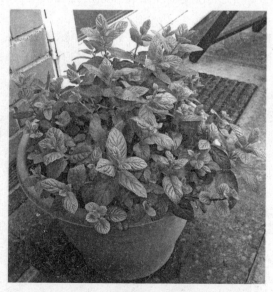

Figure 70 *Mentha spicata*, "Mint 2014-06-01 00-53"
by Sunnysingh22, own work

The confection and oral care industries consume the largest quantity of mint oil. Candy and chewing gum represent the second-largest consumer packaged goods category, second only to beer. Worldwide consumption of mint-related consumer products grew 27 percent from 1998 to 2004. The three top producers of mint oil are India, the United States, and China. High production costs have affected mint oil production. In 1997, the United States produced 6,400 metric tonnes of mint oil; in 2005, this figure dropped to 4,000 metric tonnes. India's production doubled during the same period to 1,500 metric tonnes. Most mint oil production is from *M. piperita* (peppermint), *M. spicata* (spearmint), and *M. arvensis* (Japanese mint). The following table lists the estimated worldwide production of mint oils.

Estimated worldwide production of mint oil

Species	Area (ha.)	Production (metric tonnes)	Total world production (metric tonnes)	Major producing countries
Japanese mint	60,000	12,000	16,000	India, China, Brazil
Peppermint	2,500	200	4,000	USA, France, former USSR, Brazil, India
Bergamot mint	1,200	150	200	USA, Brazil, Thailand
Spearmint	3,000	300	2,000	USA, China, former USSR, India

Source: Essential Oils Association of India (2001), Vision 2005

Ancient Egyptians used mint in the popular incense Kyphi, to flavour food and wine, and to treat gastric ailments, a cure that is still used today. Ancient Assyrians used it as incense in their rituals to the Fire God. Greeks regarded mint as a symbol of hospitality. They used it to clean their banquet tables and added it to their baths as a stimulant. Greek athletes rubbed bruised leaves on their skin after bathing, believing it increased strength. Romans and Greeks flavoured drinking water with fresh mint. Slaves were made to drink a tonic made from barley water flavoured with mint to freshen their breath.

Pliny advocated that students wear wreaths of mint to sharpen their minds. Senators wore mint sprigs to improve their oratory skills and control tempers. Pliny wrote that mint stirred the mind and appetite. Romans used mint in sauces as a digestive aid and mouth freshener. Pliny, Hippocrates, and Aristotle believed that mint discouraged sexual intercourse.

Chinese medical writings in the Tang Peng Tao period (c. 659 AD) mention mint as a treatment for stomachaches and chest pains. The herb is still used today for indigestion, common colds, and bad breath. Ancient Jews used it to freshen synagogue floors and crowded temples. Mint is referred to in the Bible as one of the tithe herbs. It is speculated that mint was one of the bitter herbs used in the Last Supper.

Europeans in the Middle Ages used the stems and leaves for insect bites, digestive problems, and to freshen drinking water on long sea voyages. Its cooling sensation was useful for treating minor burns and skin irritations. It also relieved breathing, headaches, and clogged respiratory passages. In 1790, the Altoids mint lozenge was created during the reign of King George III. These mints were made from boiled sugar and cut using a rotary tablet press, then sold throughout Europe and the United States. In 1869, Thomas Adams invented mint chewing gum. In the 1950s, a combination of mint and candy called "Certs" was produced. Then copper gluconate and cottonseed oil were combined to create a product called Restyn®, which was sold as a mouthwash and mouth freshener.

Tayarani-Najaran et al. (2013) indicate that the essential oils of both *M. spicata* and *M. piperita* have antiemetic effects in chemotherapy patients. Experiments with essential oil conducted on rats indicate that it has antitumor properties (Hajighasemi, 2011). Studies conducted by Kazemi, Rostami, and Shafiei (2012) indicate that *M. piperita* has antibacterial and antifungal activities, though less than that of *M. spicata*. Carvone possessed the highest antibacterial and antifungal activity among the tested components.

Nozhat (2014) revealed that spearmint has no significant toxic effect on the reproductive system, fertility, or number of offspring in adult male rats; however, excess amounts of spearmint tea may affect fertility. Studies indicate that spearmint reduces free testosterone levels in the blood but does not affect total testosterone and DHEA levels, a property that may help treat hirsutism in women.

Spearmint oil is said to benefit the digestive system by relieving flatulence, constipation, vomiting, and nausea, as well as respiratory tract ailments like cough, bronchitis, asthma, catarrh, and sinus. It is used to flavour confections (e.g., milkshakes, chewing gum), especially in North America, and in personal care products (e.g., toothpaste).

Peppermint essential oil gives a cooling sensation on the mucosa and skin and a calming effect on the body. It is used in aromatherapy to relieve sore muscles and headaches. It can also be added to cleaning supplies for antimicrobial power and fragrance. An organic essential oil mosquito repellent that has a blend of cinnamon, eugenol, geranium, peppermint, and lemongrass oils is also sold in the market. This use is quite similar to that practiced by the ancient Egyptians, Greeks, Romans, and Jews.

M. piperita is widely used in medicines to relieve digestive problems including heartburn, nausea, vomiting, morning sickness, irritable bowel syndrome, cramps, upset stomach, diarrhoea, liver and gall bladder complaints, spasms during endoscopy procedures, and as a stimulant. Kaushik et al. (2013) confirmed the hepatoprotective potential of alcoholic extract of *M. piperita* leaves in controlling the development of radio-lesions and abnormal hepatocytes in the liver. They attribute this protection to its antioxidant and antiperoxidant properties. Ford et al. (2008) suggest that doctors recommend peppermint oil, fiber, and antispasmodics as first-line treatments for irritable bowel syndrome. Peppermint oil can cause heartburn, however, so it is contraindicated in patients with bile duct obstruction, gallbladder inflammation, or severe liver damage.

Caution is advised in patients with gastrointestinal reflux (Longwood Herbal Task Force; http://www.longwoodherbal. org/peppermint/peppermint.pdf). Menthol products should not be used directly under the nose of small children and infants because of the risk of apnea. Peppermint is categorized as "Generally Recognized as Safe" by the U.S. FDA and has few side effects. However, in 1990, the FDA banned the sale of peppermint oil as an over-the-counter drug for use as a digestive aid, because its effectiveness had not been proven. It is now sold as a dietary supplement, and does not require FDA approval to be marketed, as it cannot claim to prevent or treat illnesses.

Iscan et al. (2002) used a bio-autography assay to show antimicrobial activity of menthol. Jayakumar et al. (2011) also found peppermint oil to possess strong broad-spectrum antibiotic activity that is comparable to some allopathic antibiotic drugs. The use of peppermint by humans was also found to be beneficial in prevention and treatment of risk factors of chronic degenerative diseases (Barbalho et al., 2011).

Results from clinical trials of homeopathic treatments show that *M. piperita* had a marked effect on the respiratory system (Chakraborty et al., 2008). Taher (2012) tested and verified the analgesic property of the oil on rats. Kligler et al. (2007) quotes two trials that demonstrate the efficacy of peppermint oil for relieving tension headache. One trial found peppermint oil to be as effective as acetaminophen (Tylenol, paracetamol).

Roussos and Hirsch (2014) found that, for people with alliaceous migraines, "Nose plug and counter stimulation with peppermint prevented the onset of headaches and associated symptoms." Alliaceous migraines are those caused by onions, garlic, and other alliums (usually the odour). Peppermint is also used for treating nausea and vomiting during pregnancy but studies to validate this property have been inconclusive or contradictory.

As modern communication, transportation, culture, and culinary habits spread across continents, and as fast food from places like Pizza Hut, McDonalds, and Kentucky Fried become popular, the diverse culinary habitats of Asia, Africa, Europe, and North and South America have changed. A new global cuisine is perhaps emerging that includes herbs and spices from all parts of the globe. Ancient herbal medicine systems from Asia, particularly Traditional Chinese Medicine and Ayurveda, are gaining popularity in the United States and Europe.

Many herbal formulations are now sold in American and European markets, mainly in the form of nutraceuticals. Herbal formulations are becoming popular in perfumes, creams, and other cosmetic products. The American Herbal Products Association includes more than 1,000 companies as members, a testament to the growing popularity of herbs in America and Canada. However, the herb industry must evolve along with modern scientific practices and processes to get approval from institutions like the U.S. FDA and other governing bodies.

In my next book, I will focus on some popular herbs, trees, and plants from Asia. Many of these herbs have been in use as food, cosmetics, and medicines in the United States and Europe, for centuries.

WRAPPING UP

⁓

Natural commodities were the mainstay for the survival of man from ancient times, until probably the last century.

During pre-industrial times, plants and herbs were the main source of food, shelter, medicine, cosmetics, and fibre. Aromatic gums and resins from plants were used in temples as incense and for personal adornment. Oil from the seeds was consumed for food, and herbs and herbal products were used in healing. Given their importance to society, plants have found their way into religious and secular thinking and literature. Post the industrial revolution, alternatives to plants have emerged, although these continue to be centre stage to human beings.

There existed up to the middle of the first millennium AD the following major ancient civilizations: India, China, Greece and Rome, Egypt, Mesopotamia, and Persia. These civilizations, in spite of existence of considerable logistical challenges, actively traded with each other.

While herbs have a universal appeal to man, it is difficult to ignore the fact that religion, regions and cultures divide the world. A book on herbs that seeks to trace the history of man perforce has to rely on literature and evidence left by man. What should be the base literature that should be used for such a work, was the question confronting me. There were a few options available.

The oldest work that has extensive references to plants came from the Yellow Emperor of China—Huangdi Neijing (2706 BC-2697 BC). We have the Rigveda, the sacred text of the Hindus that is said to have been enunciated from 1700 BC to 1100 BC, which also has extensive references to plants, trees, and herbs. But the body of research available in the public domain and in English for either of these two works, is limited.

The Bible became the natural choice. Its origin goes back to 1312 BC (others have placed this event at 1280 BC) when Moses is said to have had a revelation at Mount Sinai. The first five books of *the Bible--Genesis, Exodus, Leviticus, Numbers,* and *Deuteronomy* have extensive references to plants and herbs in use during these earlier times. Plants are also mentioned in the New Testament.

Additionally, the Bible was written in the region of ancient Israel that lay at the crossroads of lands where Judaism, Christianity, and Islam arose. Christianity and Islam together constitute the majority of humanity on earth. While the Bible is a highly researched work, most of this has been done from the point of view of faith, rather than science.

Another factor that tilted the scale in favor of using the Bible as the base for a book on herbs was the availability of a lot of other regional literature. There are works written by Greek and Roman philosophers like Hippocrates, Galen, Pliny, and many other scholars from the ancient times to this day. We have the

Ebers Papyrus which is a record of medicinal practices used by Ancient Egyptians and much more.

The Mesopotamian, Egyptian, Greek, Roman, and Persian empires imported a large quantity of herbs and spices from India, China, the islands around the Malacca Straits, and Africa. Many of these commodities were trans-shipped to Indian ports on their onward journey to the Red Sea and the Mediterranean Sea. The Bible, therefore, stands at the right spot for tracing a global history of herbs from ancient to modern times.

Even though extensive references and descriptions of plants used are available in the world, most of them have used local names. Connecting these to a universally understood scientific name is always a challenge. Identification of plants became a subjective interpretation act. I have had to fall back on my own research, field experience, and forestry training to draw conclusions on the source of many of these plants and herbs. Ecology, climate, logistics, use of plants in the place where they are still found are factors that determined the linking of a local name and my choice of their probable scientific identity.

During the course of this analysis, I observed that a herbal product could have more than one species as its source. Multiple species were analysed in detail to present a comprehensive picture of a plant and plant product. Botanists and taxonomists may find this aspect of interest. Further research on these aspects will be required before any definitive conclusions on the correct botanical species of the plants mentioned in the Bible can be made.

The absence of proper conservation strategies have led to the overexploitation of many of the popular human use herbs and their products. This has led to a rapid depletion of numbers of some species. For instance, the stately cedars of Lebanon that were extensively used in shipbuilding by the ancient Romans are now restricted to a small area of modern Lebanon.

Efforts have been made to cultivate some of the more popular of these species. In some cases like saffron, the wild stock became extinct probably at the time of the cataclysmic volcanic eruptions that covered most islands of Akrotiri in Greece in 1647 BC. Saffron is now found only as a cultivated crop.

Agroforestry and silvicultural practices have evolved over time. Some of the plants mentioned in the Bible were too valuable to be lost forever. Efforts to rejuvenate some of the crops in their natural habitats have been successful. In other cases, species have depleted and placed under threatened species category. Omani frankincense that yields the best resin is a threatened species. Agarwood is also under threat. You will find mentions of cultivation and conservation practices in the detailed descriptions of the plants. There have also been instances where chemical alternatives have been identified and the use of natural products is no longer popular.

Plants have been popular for their healing property. Even with the advancements made in modern medicine that rely substantially on chemicals for drug manufacture, plants continue to be a preferred option as supplements and as herbal medicine even today. This is an area that is debated extensively by natural product experts, doctors, scientists, and regulators. In some countries like the United States, the use of natural products as medicine is not permitted by the regulator. While there exists a constituency in the world that swear by the efficacy of medicinal use of herbal products, the larger modern medicine community continues to be circumspect.

The earliest drug discoveries were of organic origin. But soon, the drug industry found that it made business sense to shift focus and look for a more stable source. Natural products presented the challenges of consistency and reliability of raw materials supply. Chemicals were a better alternative. Soon, these became the main source for all new and existing drugs.

Dozens of scientists across the globe are working on natural products. High impact scientific journals have numerous papers documenting experiments that present the positive and negative effects of natural products on living organisms. Many trials have validated natural product based ancient remedies, too. However, most scientific literature has rarely gone beyond animal trials. Cases of human trials that have conclusively demonstrated the efficacy of natural products are too few.

Recently, Sun Pharma, an Indian pharmaceutical firm, announced a tie up with a research institution to develop a new drug to treat dengue. The drug under development is from a botanical source. There are similar efforts underway in other parts of the world.

The hunt for the next natural products based blockbuster drug generally continues to evade science. The current state of research aimed at validating medicinal use of plants has been extensively covered and referenced in this book. In most cases, the conclusions are mixed. However, the future of scientifically supported medicinal use of plants appears to be bright, even though a lot more needs to be done to accomplish this dream.

The plant kingdom is diverse and rich. It is impossible to research and present a complete and comprehensive description of all the species mentioned in the Bible. But the major species still held valuable by people across the world have been picked and the details presented in the book. The next book will describe herbs from Asia—mainly from India and China. Scholars and readers are welcome to present their views on this book on the comments page of my website—www.sudhirahluwalia.com

BIBLIOGRAPHY

CHAPTER 1 – HISTORICAL OVERVIEW

Ben-Yehoshua, S., Borowitz, C., & Hanus, L. O. *Frankincense, myrrh, and balm of Gilead: Ancient spices of Southern Arabia and Judea. In J. Janick (Ed.), Horticultural Reviews* (Vol. 39). Hoboken, NJ: John Wiley & Sons, 2011. doi: 10.1002/9781118100592.ch1

Kashyap, A., & Weber, S. *Harappan plant use revealed by starch grains from Farmana, India, Antiquity,* 2010. 84(326), 933-398.

Potts, D. T. *Mesopotamian civilization: The material foundations.* Ithaca, NY: Cornell University Press, 1997.

Saul, H., Madella, M., Fischer, A., Glykou, A., Hartz, S., & Craig, O. E., *Phytoliths in pottery reveal the use of spice in European prehistoric cuisine, PLoS ONE,* 2013, *8*(8), e70583.

CHAPTER II – HOLY ANOINTING OILS
MYRRH

Amiel, E., Ofir, R., Dudai, N., Soloway, E., Rabinsky, T., & Rachmilevitch, S. β-*Caryophyllene, a compound isolated from the biblical balm of Gilead (Commiphora gileadensis), is a selective apoptosis inducer for tumor cell lines. Evidence-Based Complementary and Alternative Medicine, 2012,* 872394. doi: 10.1155/2012/872394.

Arora, R. B., Das, D., Kapoor, S. C., & Sharma, R. C. *Effect of some fractions of Commiphora mukul on various serum lipid levels in hypercholesterolemic chicks and their effectiveness in myocardial infarction in rats, Indian Journal of Experimental Biology*, 1973. *11*(3), 166-168.

Arya, V. P. *"Gugulipid" Drugs of the Future*, 1988. 13(7), 618-619.

Baldwa, V. S., Bhasin, V., Ranka, P. C., & Mathur, K. M. *Effects of Commiphora mukul (Guggul) in experimentally induced hyperlipemia and atherosclerosis, Journal of the Association of Physicians of India*, 1981. *29*(1), 13-17.

Deng, R. *Therapeutic effects of guggul and its constituent guggulsterone: Cardiovascular benefits, Cardiovascular Drug Reviews*, 2007. *25*(4), 375-390.

Gujral, M. L., Sareen, K., Tangri, K. K., Amma, M. K., & Roy, A.K. *Antiarthritic and anti-inflammatory activity of gum guggul (Balsamodendron mukul Hook), Indian Journal of Physiology and Pharmacology*, 1960. 40, 267-273.

Hanuš, L. O., Rezanka, T., Dembitsky, V. M., & Moussaieff, A. *Myrrh—Commiphora chemistry, Biomedical papers of the Medical Faculty of the University Palacký, Olomouc, Czechoslovakia*, 2005. 149(1), 3-27.

Iluz, D., Hoffman, M., Gilboa-Garber, N., & Amar, Z. *Medicinal properties of Commiphora gileadensis, African Journal of Pharmacy and Pharmacology*, 2010. 4(8), 516-520.

Ishnava, K. B., Mahida, Y. N., & Mohan, J. S. S. *In vitro assessments of antibacterial potential of Commiphora wightii (Arn.) Bhandari. gum extract. Journal of Pharmacognosy and Phytotherapy*, 2010. 2(7), 91-96.

Kuppurajan, K., Rajagopalan, S. S., Rao, T. K., & Sitaraman, R. (1978). *Effect of guggulu (Commiphora mukul–Engl.) on serum lipids in obese, hypercholesterolemic and hyperlipemic cases. Journal of the Association of Physicians of India*, 1978. 26, 367-373.

Morteza-Semnani, K., & Saeedi, M. Constituents of the essential oil of *Commiphora myrrha* (Nees) Engl. var. *molmol. Journal of Essential Oil Research*, 2003. 1*5*(1), 50-51.

Omer, S. A., Adam, S. E. I., & Mohammed, O. B. *Antimicrobial activity of Commiphora myrrha against some bacteria and Candida albicans isolated from gazelles at King Khalid Wildlife Research Centre. Research Journal of Medicinal Plant*, 2011. 5, 65-71.

Patil, V. D., Nayak, U. R., & Dev, S. *Chemistry of Ayurvedic drugs. I. Guggulu. (a resin from Commiphora mukul) steroidal constituents. Tetrahedron*, 1972. 28, 2341.

Provan, G. J., Gray, A. I., & Waterman, P. G. *Sesquiterpenes from the myrrh type resins of some Kenyan commiphora species. Flavour and Fragrance Journal*, 1987. 2(3), 109-113.

Purushothaman, K. K., & Chandrasekharan, S. *Guggul sterols from C. mukul. Indian Journal of Chemistry*, 1976. 14, 802.

Saxena, G., Singh, S. P., Pal, R., Singh, S., Pratap, R., & Nath, C. *Gugulipid, an extract of Commiphora whighitii with lipid-lowering properties, has protective effects against streptozotocin-induced memory deficits in mice. Pharmacology Biochemistry and Behavior*, 2007, *86*(4), 797-805.

Siddiqui, M. Z., & Mazumder, P. M. Comparative study of hypolipidemic profile of resinoids of *Commiphora mukul/ Commiphora wightii* from different geographical locations. *Indian Journal of Pharmaceutical Sciences*, 2012. *74*(5), 422-427.

Singh, M., Singh, S., & Rekha Antifungal activity of *Commiphora wightii*, an important medicinal plant. *Asian Journal of Plant Science and Research*, 2013. *3*(3), 24-27.

Singh, R. B., Niaz, M. A., & Ghosh, S. *Hypolipidemic and antioxidant effects of Commiphora mukul as an adjunct to dietary therapy in patients with hypercholesterolemia. Cardiovascular Drugs Therapy*, 1994. *8*, 659-664.

Ulbricht, C., Basch, E., Szapary, P., Hammerness, P., Axentsev, S., Boon, H., . . . Woods, J. *Guggul for hyperlipidemia: A review by the Natural Standard Research Collaboration. Complementary Therapies in Medicine*, 2005. 13, 279-290.

Verma, S. K., & Bordia, A. *Effect of Commiphora mukul (gum guggulu) in patients of hyperlipidemia with special reference to HDL-cholesterol. Indian Journal of Medical Research*, 1988. *87*, 356-360.

Xu, J., Guo, Y., Zhao, P., Xie, C., Jin, D., Hou, W., & Zhang, T. (2011). Neuroprotective cadinane sesquiterpenes from the resinous exudates of *Commiphora myrrha. Fitoterapia*, *82*(8), 1198-1201.

Zaidi, S. M. A., Pathan, S. A., Ahmad, F. J., Surender, S., Jamil, S., & Khar, R. K. *Anticonvulsant and neurotoxicity profile of Commiphora gileadensis (L.) C. Chr. Planta Medica*, 2010. *76*, P84.

Zhu, N., Kikuzaki, H., Sheng, S., Sang, S., Rafi, M. M., Wang, M., . . . Ho, C. T. Furanosesquiterpenoids of *Commiphora myrrha. Journal of Natural Products*, 2001. *64*(11), 1460-1462.

CALAMUS

Abegaz, B., Yohanne, P. G., & Diete, K. R. *Constituents of the essential oil of Ethiopian Cymbopogon citratus stapf. Journal of Natural Products*, 1983. *146*, 423-426.

Adeneye, A. A., & Agbaje, E. O. *Hypoglycemic and hypolipidemic effects of fresh leaf aqueous extract of Cymbopogon citratus Stapf in rats. Journal of Ethnopharmacology*, 2007. *112*, 440-444.

Agbafor, K. N., & Akubugwo, E. I. Hypocholesterolaemic effect of ethanolic extract of fresh leaves of *Cymbopogon citratus* (lemon grass). *African Journal of Biotechnology*, 2007. *6*(5), 596-598.

Ahmad, S., Ashraf, N., Nisar-ur-Rehman, Nazir, M., Ahraf, S., Akhtar, K. S., . . . Simjee, S. U. *Anticonvulsant and antimicrobial activities of the methanolic extract of Cymbopogon jwarancusa. Journal of Tropical Medicinal Plants*, 2010. *11*(1), 39-44.

Al-Ghamdi, S. S., Al-Ghamdi, A. A., & Shammah, A. A. *Inhibition of calcium oxalate nephrotoxicity with Cymbopogon schoenanthus (Al-Ethkher). Drug Metabolism Letters*, 2007. *1*(4), 241-244.

Amina, R. M., Aliero, B. L., & Gumi, A. M. *Phytochemical screening and oil yield of a potential herb, camel grass (Cymbopogon schoenanthus* Spreng.). *Central European Journal of Experimental Biology*, 2013. *2*(3), 15-19.

Blanco, M. M., Costa, C. A., Freire, A. O., Santos, J. G., & Costa, I. M. *Neurobehavioral effect of essential oil of Cymbopogon citratus in mice. Phytomedicine*, 2007. *16*(2-3), 265-270.

Bose, S. C, Ammani, K., & Ratakumari, S. *Chemical composition and its antibacterial activity of essential oil from Cymbopoton jwarancusa. International Journal of Biopharmaceutical Research*, 2013. *2*(2), 97-100.

Buch, P., Patel, V., Ranpariya, V., Sheth, N., & Parmar, S. *Neuroprotective activity of Cymbopogon martinii against cerebral ischemia/ reperfusion-induced oxidative stress in rats. Journal of Ethnopharmacology*, 2012. *142*(1), 35-40.

Caballero-Gallardo, K., Olovero-Verbel, J., & Stashenko, E. E. *Repellency and toxicity of essential oils from Cymbopogon martinii, Cymbopogon flexuosus*and *Lippia origanoides* cultivated in Colombia against *Tribolium castaneum. Journal of Stored Products Research*, 2012. *50*, 62-65.

Carbajal, D., Casaco, A., Arruzazabala, L., Gonzalez, R., & Tolon, Z. *Pharmacological study of Cymbopogon citratus leaves. Journal of Ethnopharmacology*, 1989. *25*(1), 103-107.

Cavalcanti, E. S., Morais, S. M., & Lima, M. A. *Larvicidal activity of essential oils from Brazilian plants against Aedes aegypti L. Memórias do Instituto Oswaldo Cruz*, 2004. *99*(5), 541-544.

Chandan, P., Digvijay, S., & Omkar, S. *Study of antimicrobial activity and carbon composition by GC-FID of extract from Cymbopogon jwarancusa* (Jones.) *International Journal of Natural Products Research*, 2013. *3*(3), 57-61.

Cheel, J., Theoduloz, C., Rodriäguez, J., & Hirschmann, S. G. *Free radical scavengers and antioxidants from lemongrass (Cymbopogon citratus (DC.) Stapf.). Journal of Agricultural and Food Chemistry*, 2005. *53*(7), 2511-2517.

D'Souza, A. M., Paknikar, S. K., Dev, V., Beauchamp, P. S., & Kamat, S. P. *Biogenetic-type synthesis of (+)-cymbodiacetal, a constituent of Cymbopogon martini. Journal of Natural Products*, 2004. *67*(4), 700-702.

Devi, R. C., Sim, S. M., & Ismail, R. Effect of *Cymbopogon citratus and citral on vascular smooth muscle of the isolated thoracic rat aorta. Evidence-Based Complementary and Alternative Medicine*, 2012. 539475. doi:10.1155/2012/539475.

Gacche, R. N., Shaikh, R. U., Chapole, S. M., Jadhav, A. D., & Jadhav, S. G. *Kinetics of inhibition of monoamine oxidase using Cymbopogon martinii (Roxb.) Wats.: A potential antidepressant herbal ingredient with antioxidant activity. Indian Journal of Clinical Biochemistry*, 2011. *26*(3), 303-308.

Gbenou, J. D., Ahounou, J. F., Akakpo, H. B., Laleye, A., Yayi, E., Gbaguidi, F., . . . Kotchoni, S. O. *Phytochemical composition of Cymbopogon citratus and Eucalyptus citriodora essential oils and their anti-inflammatory and analgesic properties on Wistar rats. Molecular Biology Reports*, 2013. *40*(2), 1127-1134.

Ghosh, M. *Antifungal properties of haem peroxidase from Acorus calamus. Annals of Botany*, 2006. *98*(6), 1145-1153.

Gilani, A. U., Shah, A. J., Ahmad, M., & Shaheen, F. *Antispasmodic effect of Acorus calamus Linn. is mediated through calcium channel blockade. Phytotherapy Research*, 2006. *20*(12), 1080-1084.

Guanasingh, C. B., & Nagarajan, S. *Flavonoids of Cymbopogon citratus. Indian Journal of Pharmaceutical Science*, 1981. *43*, 115.

Hanson, S. W., Crawford, M., Koker, M. E. S., & Menezes, F. A. *Cymbopogonol, a new triterpenoid from Cymbopogon citratus. Phytochemistry*, 1976. *15*(6), 1074-1075.

Hu, B. Y., & Ji, Y. Y. *Research on the anticarcinogenic activation of Acorus calcamus. Anticarcinogenic activation of alpha-asarone on human carcinoma cells. Zhong Xi Yi Jie He Za Zhi*, 1986. *6*(8), 480-483, 454.

Imam, H., Riaz, Z., Azhar, M., Sofi, G., & Hussain, A. *Sweet flag (Acorus calamus Linn.): An incredible medicinal herb. International Journal of Green Pharmacy*, 7, 2013. 288-296.

Katiki, L. M., Chagas, A. C., Takahira, R. K., Juliani, H. R., Ferreira, J. F., & Amarante, A. F. *Evaluation of Cymbopogon schoenanthus essential oil in lambs experimentally infected with Haemonchus contortus. Veterinary Parasitology*, 2012. *186*(3-4), 312-318.

Ketoh, G. K., Koumaglo, H. K., Glitho, I. A., & Huignard, J. *Comparative effects of Cymbopogon schoenanthus essential oil and piperitone on Callosobruchus maculatusdevelopment. Fitoterapia*, 2006. *77*(7-8), 506-510.

Khadhri, A., Mokni, R. E. I., Araújo, M. E. M. *Screening of the antimicrobial properties of the essential oils of Cymbopogon schoenanthus. Tropical Journal of Medical Research*, 2011. *15*(2).

Khadri, A., Neffati, M., Smiti, S., Falé, P., Lino, A. R. L., Serralheiro, M. L. M., & Araújo, M. E. M. *Antioxidant, antiacetylcholinesterase and antimicrobial activities of Cymbopogon schoenanthus L. Spreng (lemon grass) from Tunisia. LWT - Food Science and Technology*, 2010. *43*(2), 331-336.

Lawrence, K., Lawrence, R., Parihar, D., Srivastava, R., & Charan, A. *Antioxidant activity of palmarosa essential oil (Cymbopogon martini) grown in north Indian plains. Asian Pacific Journal of Tropical Disease*, 2012. *2*(2), S888-S891.

Leite, J. R., Seabra, M. L., Maluf, E., Assolant, K., Suchecki, D., Tufik, S., . . . Carlini, E. A. *Pharmacology of lemongrass (Cymbopogon citratus Stapf). III. Assessment of eventual toxic, hypnotic and anxiolytic effects on humans. Journal of Ethnopharmacology*, 1986. *17*(1), 75-83.

Marongiu, B., Piras, A., Porcedda, S., & Tuveri, E. *Comparative analysis of the oil and supercritical CO(2) extract of Cymbopogon citratus Stapf. Natural Product Research*, 2006. *20*(5), 455-459.

Matouschek, B. K., & Stahl, B. E. *Phytochemical study of non-volatile substances from Cymbopogon citratus (DC.) Stapf (Poaceae). Pharmaceutica Acta Helvetiae*, 1991. *66*, 242-245.

Meevatee, U., Boontim, S., Keereeta, O., Vinitketkumnuen, U., & O-ariyakul, N. (1993). *Antimutagenic activity of lemon grass. In Boot-in, S (Ed.) Man and Environment.* Chiang Mai, Thailand: Chiang Mai. University Press, 1993.

Motley, T. J. *The ethnobotany of sweet flag, Acorusc alamusl* (araceae). *Economic Botany*, 1994. *48*(4), 397-412.

Nallamuthu, I., Singsit, D., & Khanum, F. *Effect of rhizome extract of Acorus calamus on depressive condition induced by forced swimming in mice. International Journal of Phytomedicine*, 2012. *4*(3), 319-325.

Nambiar, V. S., & Matela, H. *Potential functions of lemon grass (Cymbopogon citratus) in health and disease. International Journal of Pharmaceutical & Biological Archives*, 2012. *3*(5), 1035-1043.

Onawunmia, G. O., Yisak, W. A., & Ogunlana, E. O. *Antibacterial constituents in the essential oil of Cymbopogon citratus (DC.) Stapf. Journal of Ethnopharmacology*, 1984. *12*, 279-286.

Othman, M. B., Han, J., El Omri, A., Ksouri, R., Neffati, M., & Isoda, H. *Antistress effects of the ethanolic extract from Cymbopogon schoenanthus growing wild in Tunisia. Evidence-Based Complementary and Alternative Medicine*, 2013. 737401.

Puatanachokchai, R. *Antimutagenicity, cytotoxicity and antitumor activity from lemon grass (Cymbopogon citratus, Stapf) extract (Unpublished master's thesis).* Chiang Mai University, Thailand, 1994.

Puatanachokchai, R., Kishida, H., Denda, A., Murata, N., Konishi, Y., Vinitketkumnuen, U., & Nakae, D. *Inhibitory effects of lemon grass (Cymbopogon citratus, Stapf) extract on the early phase of hepatocarcinogenesis after initiation with ethylnitrosamine in male Fischer 344 rats. Cancer Letters*, 2002. *183*(1), 9-15.

Prasad, C., Singh, D., & Shukla, O. *Antioxidant activity and trace elements profile of extracts of Cymbopogon jwarancusa (Jones.) leaves. Journal of Pharmacognosy and Phytochemistry*, 2013. *2*(3), 33-37.

Radušienė, J., Judžentienė, A., Pečiulytė, D., & Janulis, V. *Essential oil composition and antimicrobial assay of Acorus calamus leaves from different wild populations. Plant Genetic Resources: Characterization and Utilization*, 2007. *5*, 37-44.

Ratti, N., Kumar, S., Verma, H. N., & Gautam, S. P. *Improvement in bioavailability of tricalcium phosphate to Cymbopogon martinii var. motia by rhizobacteria, AMF and Azospirillum inoculation. Microbiology Research*, 2001. *156*(2), 145-149.

Shah, A. J., & Gilani, A. H. *Blood pressure-lowering and vascular modulator effects of Acorus calamus extract are mediated through multiple pathways. Journal of Cardiovascular Pharmacology*, 2009. *54*(1), 38-46.

Shah, G., Shri, R., Panchal, V., Sharma, N., Singh, B., & Mann, A. S. *Scientific basis for the therapeutic use of Cymbopogon citratus, stapf (Lemon grass). Journal of Advanced Pharmaceutical Technology and Research,* 2011. *2*(1), 3-8.

Shukla, P. K., Khanna, V. K., Ali, M. M., Maurya, R., Khan, M. Y., & Srimal, R. C. *Neuroprotective effect of Acorus calamus against middle cerebral artery occlusion-induced ischaemia in rat. Human and Experimental Toxicology,* 2006. *25*(4), 187-194.

Siddiqui, N., & Garg, S. C. *Chemical composition of Cymbopogon martinii (Roxb.) Wats. var. martinii. Journal of Essential Oil Research,* 1990. *2*(2), 93-94.

Sonker, N., Pandey, A. K., Singh, P., & Tripathi, N. N. *Assessment of Cymbopogon citratus (DC.) Stapf essential oil as herbal preservatives based on antifungal, antiaflatoxin, and antiochratoxin activities and in vivo efficacy during storage. Journal of Food Science,* 2014. *79*(4), M628–M634.

Sousa, S. M., Silva, P. S., & Viccini, L. F. *Cytogenotoxicity of Cymbopogon citratus (DC) Stapf (lemon grass) aqueous extracts in vegetal test systems. Anais da Academia Brasileira de Ciências*, 2010. *82*(2), 305-311.

Souza-Formigoni, M. L., Lodder, H. M., Gianotti, F. O., Ferreira, T. M., & Carlini, E. A. *Pharmacology of lemongrass (Cymbopogon citratus Stapf). II. Effects of daily two month administration in male and female rats and in offspring exposed "in utero". Journal of Ethnopharmacology,* 1986. *17*(1), 65-74.

Suaeyun, R., Kinouchi, T., Arimochi, H., Vinitketkumnuen, U., & Ohnishi, Y. *Inhibitory effects of lemon grass (Cymbopogon citratus Stapf) on formation of azoxymethane-induced DNA adducts and aberrant crypt foci in the rat colon. Carcinogenesis,* 1997. *18*, 949-955.

Tiwari, R. K. S., Das, K., Pandey, D., Tiwari, R. B., & Dubey, J. *Rhizome Yield of Sweet Flag (Acorus calamus L.) as influenced by planting season, harvest time, and spacing. International Journal of Agronomy,* 2012. 731375.

Vinitketkumnuen, U., Puatanachokchai, R., Kongtawelert, P., Lertprasertsuke, N., & Matsushima, T. *Antimutagenicity of lemon grass (Cymbopogon citratus, Stapf) to various known mutagens in salmonella mutation assay. Mutation Research,* 1994. *341*(1), 71-75.

Vohora, S. B., Shah, S. A., & Dandiya, P. C. *Central nervous system studies on an ethanol extract of Acorus calamus rhizomes. Journal of Ethnopharmacology,* 1990. *28*(1), 53-62.

Wannissorn, B., Jarikasem, S., & Soontorntanasart, T. *Antifungal activity of lemon grass and lemon grass oil cream. Phytotherapy Research,* 1996. *10*, 551-554.

CINNAMON

Al-Dhubiab, B. E. *Pharmaceutical applications and phytochemical profile of Cinnamomum burmannii. Pharmacognosy Reviews,* 2012.*6*(12), 125-131.

Chan, L. Y. *Bioassay-guided purification and characterization of anti-inflammatory components in Cinnamomum burmannii (Unpublished senior thesis).* University of Wisconsin-Madison, USA, 2010.

Daker, M., Lin, V. Y., Akowuah, G. A., Yam, M. F., & Ahmad, M. *Inhibitory effects of Cinnamomum burmannii Blume stem bark extract and trans-cinnamaldehyde on nasopharyngeal carcinoma cells; synergism with cisplatin. Experimental and Theoretical Medicine,* 2013. *5*(6), 1701-1709.

Huang, S., Pan, Y., Gan, D., Ouyang, X., Tang, S., Ekunwe, S. I. N., & Wang, H. *Antioxidant activities and UV-protective properties of melanin from the berry of Cinnamomum burmannii and Osmanthus fragrans. Medicinal Chemistry Research*, 2011. *20*(4), 475-481.

Islam, R., Khan, R. I., Al-Reza, S. M., Jeong, Y. T., Song, C. H., & Khalequzzaman, M. *Chemical composition and insecticidal properties of Cinnamomum aromaticum (Nees) essential oil against the stored product beetle Callosobruchus maculatus (F.). Journal of the Science of Food and Agriculture*, 2009. *89*, 1241-1246. doi: 10.1002/jsfa.3582.

Khatib, A., Kim, M. Y., & Chung, S. K. *Anti-inflammatory activities of Cinnamomum burmanni B1. Food Science and Biotechnology*, 2005. *14*, 223-227.

Lisawati, Y., & Sulianti, S. B. *The influence of distillation time and powder size on the cinnamylaldehyde content of the volatile oil of bark of Cinnamomum burmanii Nees ex. Bl. Farmasi Indonesia*, 2002. *13*, 123-132.

Ranasinghe, P., Jayawardana, R., Galappaththy, P., Constantine, G. R., de Vas Gunawardana, N., & Katulanda, P. *Efficacy and safety of 'true' cinnamon (Cinnamomum zeylanicum) as a pharmaceutical agent in diabetes: A systematic review and meta-analysis. Diabetes Medicine*, 2012. *29*(12), 1480-1492.

Ranasinghe, P., Pigera, S., Premakurmara, G. A. S., Galappaththy, P., Constantine, G. R., & Katulanda, P. *Medicinal properties of 'true' cinnamon (Cinnamomum zeylanicum): A systematic review. BMC Complementary and Alternative Medicine*, 2013. *13*, 275.

Shan, B., Cai, Y. Z., Brooks, J. D., & Corke, H. *Antibacterial properties and major bioactive components of cinnamon stick (Cinnamomum burmannii): Activity against foodborne pathogenic bacteria. Journal of Agricultural and Food Chemistry*, 2007. *55*(14), 5484-5490.

CASSIA

Liu, J., Peter, K., Shi, D., Zhang, L., Dong, G., Zhang, D., . . . Ma, Y. Traditional formula, modern application: Chinese medicine formula Sini Tang improves early ventricular remodeling and cardiac function after myocardial infarction in rats. *Evidence-Based Complementary and Alternative Medicine*, 2014. 141938.

Sun, H., Li, T. J., Sun, L. N., Qui, Y., Huang, B. B., Yi, B., & Chen, W. S. *Inhibitory effect of traditional Chinese medicine Zi-Shen pill on benign prostatic hyperplasia in rats. Journal of Ethnopharmacology*, 2008. *115*(2), 203-208.

Yang, C-H., Li, R-X., & Chuang, L-Y. *Antioxidant activity of various parts of Cinnamomum cassia extracted with different extraction methods. Molecules*, 2012. *17*, 7294-7304.

Yu, Y-B., Dosanjh, L., Lao, L., Tan, M., Shim, B. S., & Luo, Y. *Cinnamomum cassiabark in two herbal formulas increases life span in Caenorhabditis elegans via insulin signaling and stress response pathways. PLoS ONE*, 2010. *5*(2), e9339.

CHAPTER III – INCENSES AND PERFUMES
ALOES- Aquilaria sps

Antonopoulou, M., Compton, J., Perry, L. S., & Al-Mubarak, R. *The trade and use of agarwood (Oudh) in the United Arab Emirates.* Petaling Jaya, Selangor, Malaysia: TRAFFIC Southeast Asia, 2010.

Buckingham, J. S. *Travels in Mesopotamia: Including a journey from Aleppo to Bagdad, by route of Beer, Orfah, Diatbekr, Mardin & Mousul: With researches on the ruins of Nineveh, Babylon, and other ancient cities. Vol. 2.* London: H. Colburn, 1827.

Dash, M., Patra, J. K., & Panda, P. P. *Phytochemical and antimicrobial screening of extracts of Aquilaria agallocha Roxb. African Journal of Biotechnology*, 2008. *7*(20), 3531-3534.

Fausset, A. R. *An Englishman's critical and expository Bible cyclopaedia.* London: Hodder and Stoughton, 1878.

Fu, J. L. *The Culture of Chinese Incense.* Ji'nan, China: QiLu Press, 2008.

Huang, J. Q. Wei, J. H., Zhang, Z., Yang, Y., Liu, Y. Y., Meng, H., . . . Zhang, J. L. *[Historical records and modern studies on agarwood production method and overall agarwood production method].* Zhongguo Zhong Yao Za, 2013. Zhi, *38*(3), 302-306.

Kim, Y. C., Lee, E. H., Lee, Y. M., Kim, H. K., Song, B. K., Lee, E. J., & Kim, H. M. *Effect of the aqueous extract of Aquilaria agallocha stems on the immediate hypersensitivity reactions. Journal of Ethanopharmacology,* 1997. *58*(1), 31-38.

Liu, Y., Chen, H., Yang, Y., Zhang, Z., Wei, J., Meng, H., . . . Chen, H. *Whole-tree agarwood-inducing technique: An efficient novel technique for producing high-quality agarwood in cultivated Aquilaria sinensis trees. Molecules,* 2013. *18*(3), 3086-3106.

Mao, Y-C., Hsu, H-Y., & Chiu, Y-H. *Anti-inflammatory effects and immunomodulatory mechanism of Aquilaria agallocha. Poster. 7th Asia Pacific Conference on Clinical Nutrition.* June 5-8, 2011, Bangkok, Thailand. 2011.

Miniyar, P. B., Chitre, T. S., Deuskar, H. J., Karve, S. S., & Jain, K. S. *Antioxidant activity of ethyl acetate extract of Aquilaria agallocha on nitrite-induced methaemoglobin formation. International Journal of Green Pharmacy Year,* 2008. *2*(2), 116-117.

Vakati, K., Rahman, H., Eswaraiah, M. C., & Dutta, A. M. *Evaluation of hepatoprotective activity of ethanolic extract of Aquilaria agallocha leaves (EEAA) against CCl4 induced hepatic damage in rat. Scholars Journal Applied Medical Sciences,* 2013. *1*(1), 9-12.

FRANKINCENSE- Boswellia sps

Abdel-Tawab, M., Werz, O., & Schubert-Zsilavecz, M. *Boswellia serrata: An overall assessment of in vitro, preclinical, pharmacokinetic and clinical data. Clinical Pharmacokinetics,* 2011. *50*(6), 349-369.

Abdoul-latif, F. M., Obame, L-C., Bassolé, I. H. N., & Dicko, M. H. *Antimicrobial activities of essential oil and methanol extract of Boswellia sacra Flueck. and Boswellia papyrifera (Del.) Hochst from Djibouti. International Journal of Management, Modern Sciences and Technologies*, 2012. *1*(1), 1-10.

Adake, P., Chandrashekar, R., & Rao S. N. *Potentiating antidepressant action of Boswellia serrata in acute models of depression: A preclinical study. Indo American Journal of Pharmaceutical Research*, 2013. *3*(6), 4408-4412.

Ahmed, M., Al-Daghri, N., Alokail, M. S., & Hussain, T. *Potential changes in rat spermatogenesis and sperm parameters after inhalation of Boswellia papyrifera and Boswellia carterii incense. International Journal of Environmental Research and Public Health*, 2013. *10*, 830-844.

Al Harrassi, A., Ali, L., Ceniviva, E., Al-Rawahi, A., Hussain, J., Hussain, H., . . . Al-Harrasi, R. *Antiglycation and antioxidant activities and HPTLC analysis of Boswellia sacra oleogum resin: The sacred frankincense. Tropical Journal of Pharmaceutical Research*, 2013. *12*(4), 597.

Atta-ur-Rahman, Naz, H., Fadimatou, Makhmoor, T., Yasin, A., Fatima, N., . . . Choudhary, M. I. Bioactive constituents from *Boswellia papyrifera. Journal of Natural Products*, 2005. *68*(2), 189-193.

Bekana, D., Kebede, T., Assefa, M., & Kassa, H. *Comparative phytochemical analyses of resins of Boswellia species (B. papyrifera (Del.) Hochst., B. neglecta S. Moore, and B. rivae Engl.) from northwestern, Southern, and Southeastern Ethiopia. ISRN Analytical Chemistry*, 2014. 374678.

Blain, E. J., Ali, A. Y., & Duance, V. C. *Boswellia frereana* (frankincense) *suppresses cytokine-induced matrix metalloproteinase expression and production of pro-inflammatory molecules in articular cartilage. Phytotherapy Research*, 2010. *24*(6), 905-912.

Boswellia serrata. Alternative Medicine Review, 2008. *13*(2), 165-167.

Chiavari, G., Galletti, G. C., Piccaglia, R., & Mohamud, M. A. *Differentiation between resins Boswellia carterii and Boswellia frereana (Frankincense) of Somali origin. Journal of Essential Oil Research, 1991.* 3(3), 185-186.

Demiray, H., Dereboylu, A. E., Yazici, Z. I., & Karabey, F. *Identification of benzoin obtained from calli of Styrax officinalis by HPLC. Turkish Journal of Botany*, 2013. 37(3), 956-963.

El-Nagerabi, S. A. F., Elshafie, A. E., AlKhanjari, S. S., Al-Bahry, S. N., & Elamin, M. R. *Biological activities of Boswellia sacra extracts on the growth and aflatoxins secretion of two aflatoxigenic species of Aspergillus species. Food Control*, 2013. 34(2), 763-769.

Eross, E. J. *The efficacy of Gliacin®, a derivative of Boswellia serrata extract on indomethacin responsive headache syndromes. Headache*, 2011. 51(Suppl 1), 75-76.

Farshchi, A., Ghiasi, G., Farshchi, S., & Khatabi, P. M. Effects of *Boswellia papyrifera* gum extract on learning and memory in mice and rats. *Iran Journal of Basic Medical Science*, 2010. 13(2), 9-15.

Fung, K. M., Suhail, M. M., McClendon, B., Woolley, C. L., Young, D. G., & Lin, H. K. *Management of basal cell carcinoma of the skin using frankincense (Boswellia sacra) essential oil: A case report. OA Alternative Medicine*, 2013. 1(2), 14.

Gebrehiwot, K., Muys, B., Haile, M., & Mitloehner, R. *Introducing Boswellia papyrifera (Del.) hochst and its non-timber forest product, frankincense. 7th World Forestry Congress,* Quèbec City, Canada, 2003.

Hamidpour, R., Hamidpour, S., Hamidpour, M., & Shahlari, M. Frankincense (乳香 Rû Xiāng; *Boswellia* Species): *From the selection of traditional applications to the novel phytotherapy for the prevention and treatment of serious diseases. Journal of Traditional Complement Medicine,* 2013. 3(4), 221-226.

Hasson, S. S., Al-Balushi, M. S., Sallam, T. A., Idris, M. A., Habbal, O., & Al-Jabri, A. A. *In vitro antibacterial activity of three* medicinal plants-Boswellia (Luban) species. Asian Pacific Journal of Tropical Biomedicine, 2011. 1(Suppl 2), S178-S182.

Hussain, H., Al-Harrasi, A., Al-Rawahi, A., & Hussain, J. Chemistry and biology of essential oils of genus boswellia. Evidence-Based Complementary and Alternative Medicine, 2013. 140509.

Ibrahim, M., Uddin, K. Z., & Narasu, M. L. Hepatoprotective activity of Boswellia serrata extracts: In vitro and in vivo studies. International Journal of Pharmaceutical Applications, 2011. 2(1), 89-98.

Lu, M., Xia, L., Hua, H., & Jing, Y. Acetyl-keto-beta-boswellic acid induces apoptosis through a death receptor 5-mediated pathway in prostate cancer cells. Cancer Research, 2008. 68(4), 1180-1186.

Mahmoudi, A., Hosseini-Sharifabad, A., Monsef-Esfahani, H. R., Yazdinejad, A. R., Khanavi, M., Roghani, A., . . . Sharifzadeh, M. Evaluation of systemic administration of Boswellia papyrifera extracts on spatial memory retention in male rats. Journal of Natural Medicines, 2011. 65(3-4), 519-525.

Mishra, N. K., Bstia, S., Mishra, G., Chowdary, K. A., & Patra, S. Anti-arthritic activity of Glycyrrhiza glabra, Boswellia serrata and their synergistic activity in combined formulation studied in Freund's adjuvant induced arthritic rats. Journal of Pharmaceutical Education and Research, 2011. 2(2), 92-98.

Molla, F., Gebra-Mariam, T., & Belete, A. Evaluation of local olibanum resin (Boswellia papyrifera) as microencapsulating agent for controlled release of Diclofenac sodium: Formulation, evaluation and optimization study. Pharmaceutica Analytica Acta, 2014. 5(3), 116.

Moncivaiz, A. Boswellia (Indian Frankincense). Healthline, 2013. (www.healthline.com).

Park, B., Prasad, S., Yadav, V., Sung, B., Aggarwal, B. B. Boswellic acid suppresses growth and metastasis of human pancreatic tumors in an orthotopic nude mouse model through modulation of multiple targets. PLoS One, 2011. 6(10), e26943.

Sabra, S. M. M., & Al-Masoudi, L. M. R. The effect of using

frankincense (Boswellia sacra) chewing gum on the microbial contents of buccal/oral cavity, Taif, KSA. IOSR Journal of Dental and Medical Sciences, 2014. *13*(4), 77-82.

Sedighi, B., Pardakhty, A., Kamali, H., Shafiee, K., & Hasani, B. *Effect of Boswellia papyrifera on cognitive impairment in multiple sclerosis. Iranian Journal of Neurology*, 2014. *13*(3), 149-153.

Sharma, A., Bhatia, S., Kharya, M. D., Gajbhiye, V., Ganesh, N., Namdeo, A. G., & Mahadik, K. R. *Anti-inflammatory and analgesic activity of different fractions of Boswellia serrata. International Journal of Phytomedicine*, 2010. *2*, 94-99.

Sharma, A., Chhikara, S., Ghodekar, S. N., Bhatia, S., Kharya, M. D., Gajbhiye, V., . . . Mahadik, K. R. *Phytochemical and Pharmacological investigations on Boswellia serrata. Pharmacognosy Review*, 2009. *3*(5), 206-215.

Siddiqui, M. Z. *Boswellia serrata, a potential antiinflammatory agent: An overview. Indian Journal of Pharmaceutical Science*, 2011.*73*(3), 255-261.

Singh, P., Chacko, K. M., Aggarwal, M. L., Bhat, B., Khandal, R. K., Sultana, S., & Kuruvilla, B. T. *A-90 day gavage safety assessment of Boswellia serrata in rats. Toxicology International*, 2012. *19*(3), 273-278.

Sontakke, S., Thawani, V., Pimpalkhute, S., Kabra, P., Babhulkar, S., & Hingorani, L. *Open, randomized, controlled clinical trial of Boswellia serrata extract as compared to valdecoxib in osteoarthritis of knee. Indian Journal of Pharmacology*, 2007. *39*(1), 27-29.

Strappaghetti, G., Corsano, S., Craveiroa, A., & Proietti, G. *Constituents of essential oil of Boswellia frereana. Phytochemistry*, 1982. *21*(8), 2114-2115.

Suhail, M. M., Wu, W., Cao, A., Mondalek, F. G., Fung, K. M., Shih, P. T., . . . Lin, H. K. *Boswellia sacraessential oil induces tumour cell-specific apoptosis and suppresses tumour aggressiveness in cultured human breast cancer cells. BMC Complementary Alternative Medicine*, 2011. *11*, 129.

Tole, M., Menger, D., Sass-Klaassen, U., Sterck, F. J., Copini, Pa., & Bongers, F. *Resin secretory structures of Boswellia papyrifera and implications for frankincense yield. Annals of Botany*, 2012. doi: 10.1093/aob/mcs236.

Vardar, Y., & Oflas, S. *Preliminary studies on the Styrax oil. Qualitas Plantarum et Materiae Vegetabiles*, 1973. *22*(2), 145-148.

Yadav, V. R., Prasad, S., Sung, B., Gelovani, J. G., Guha, S., Krishnan, S., & Aggarwal, B. B. *Boswellic acid inhibits growth and metastasis of human colorectal cancer in orthotopic mouse model by down regulating inflammatory, proliferative, invasive and angiogenic biomarkers. International Journal of Cancer*, 2012. *130*(9), 2176-2184.

Zhang, Y., Ning, Z., Lu, C., Zhao, S., Wang, J., Liu, B., . . . Liu, Y. *Triterpenoid resinous metabolites from the genus Boswellia: pharmacological activities and potential species-identifying properties. Chemistry Central Journal*, 2013. *7*(1) 153.

Ziyaurrahman, A. R., & Patel, J. *Anticonvulsant effect of Boswellia serrata by modulation of endogenous biomarkers. Der Pharmacia Lettre*, 2012. *4*(4), 1308-1325.

GALBANUM

Airi, S., Rawal, R. S., Dhar, U., & Purohit, A. N. *Assessment of availability and habitat preference of Jatamansi: A critically endangered medicinal plant of west Himalaya. Current Science*, 2000. *79*(10), 1467-1471.

Ebrahimzadeh, M. A., Nabavi, S. M., Nabavi, S. F., & Dehpour, A. A. *Antioxidant activity of hydroalcholic extract of Ferula gummosa Boiss roots. European Review for Medical and Pharmacological Sciences*, 2011. *15*(6), 658-664.

Eftekhar, F., Yousefzadi, M., & Borhani, K. *Antibacterial activity of the essential oil from Ferula gummosa seed. Fitoterapia*, 2004.*75*(7-8), 758-759.

Nabavi, S. F., *Ferula gummosaBoiss as a rich source of natural antioxidants with numerous therapeutic uses - A short review. In A. Capasso (Ed.), Medicinal plants as antioxidant agents: Understanding their mechanism of action and therapeutic efficacy* (15-26). Research Signpost, Trivandrum, 2012.

Sadraei, H., Asghari, G. R., Hajhashemi, V., Kolagar, A., & Ebrahimi, M. *Spasmolytic activity of essential oil and various extracts of Ferula gummosa Boiss. on ileum contractions. Phytomedicine,* 2001. *8*(5), 370-376.

Sayyah, M., Kamalinejad, M., Hidage, R. B., & Rustaiyan, A. *Antiepileptic potential and composition of the fruit essential oil of Ferula gummosa* boiss. *Iranian Biomedical Journal,* 2001. *5*(2-3), 69-72.

Sayyah, M., & Mandgary, A. *Anticonvulsant effect of Ferula gummosa root extract against experimental seizures. Iranian Biomedical Journal,* 2003. *7*(3), 139-143.

SPIKENARD

Ali, S., Ansari, K. A., Jafry, M. A., Kabeer, H., & Diwakar, G. *Nardostachys jatamansi protects against liver damage induced by thioacetamide in rats. Journal of Ethnopharmacology,* 2000. *71*(3), 359-363.

Bagchi, A., Oshima, Y., & Hikino, H. Jatamols A and B: *Sesquiterpenoids of Nardostachys jatamansi roots. Planta Medica,* 1991. *57*(3), 282-283.

Bagchi, A., Oshima, Y., & Hikino, H. *Spirojatomol, a new skeletal sesquiterpenoid of Nardostachys jatamansi roots. Tetrahedron,* 1990. *46*(5), 1523-1530.

Chatterjee, A., Basak, B., Saha, M., Dutta, U., Mukhopadhyay, C., Banerji, J., . . . Harigaya, Y. *Structure and stereochemistry of nardostachysin, a new terpenoid ester constituent of the rhizomes of Nardostachys jatamansi. Journal of Natural Products,* 2000. *63*(11), 1531-1533.

Dixit, V. P., Jain, P., & Joshi, S. C. (1988). Hypolipidaemic effects of *Curcuma longa* L and *Nardostachys jatamansi*, DC in triton-induced hyperlipidaemic rats. *Indian Journal of Physiology and Pharmacology, 32*(4), 299-304.

Gottumukkala, V. R., Annamalai, T., & Mukhopadhyay, T. *Phytochemical investigation and hair growth studies on the rhizomes of Nardostachys jatamansi* DC. *Pharmacognosy Magazine*, 2011. *7*(26), 146-150.

Hoerster, H., Ruecker, G., Tautges. *Valeranone content in the roots of Nardostachys jatamansi and Valeriana officinalis. Phytochemistry*, 1977. *16*, 1070-1071.

Lyle, N., Bhattacharyya, D., Sur, T. K., Munshi, S., Paul, P., Chatterjee, S., & Gomes, A. *Stress modulating antioxidant effect of Nardostachys jatamansi. Indian Journal of Biochemistry and Biophysics*, 2009. *46*(1), 93-98.

Metkar, B., Pal, S. C., Kasture, V., & Kasture, S. *Antidepressant activity of Nardostachys jatamansi DC. Indian Journal of Natural Products*, 1999. *15*, 10-13.

Mishra, D., Chaturvedi, R. V., & Tripathi, S. C. *The fungitoxic effect of the essential oil of the herb Nardostachys jatamansi* DC. *Tropical Agriculture*, 1995. *72*, 48-52.

Prabhu, V., Karanth, K. S., & Rao, A. (1994). Effects of *Nardostachys jatamansi* on biogenic amines and inhibitory amino acids in the rat brain. *Planta Medica, 60*(2), 114-117.

Rucker, G., Tautges, J., Sieck, A., Wenzl, H., & Graf, E. *Isolation and pharmacodynamic activity of the sesquiterpene valeranone from Nardostachys jatamansi DC [in German]. Arzneimittelforschung*, 1978. *28*(1), 7-13.

Salim, S., Ahmad, M., Zafar, K. S., Ahmad, A. S., & Islam, F. *Protective effect of Nardostachys jatamansi in rat cerebral ischemia. Pharmacology Biochemistry Behavior*, 2003. *74*(2), 481-486.

Shanbhag, S. N., Mesta, C. K., Maheshwari, M. L., Paknikar, S. K., & Bhattacharyya, S.C. *Terpenoids—LII: Jatamansin, a new terpenic coumarin from Nardostachys jatamansi. Tetrahedron*, 1964. *20*(11), 2605-2615.

SAFFRON

Abdullaev, F. I. *Cancer chemopreventive and tumoricidal properties of saffron (Crocus sativus L.). Experimental Biology and Medicine (Maywood)*, 2002. *227*(1), 20-25.

Abe, K., & Saito, H. *Effects of saffron extract and its constituent crocin on learning behaviour and long-term potentiation. Phytotherapy Research*, 2000. *14*(3), 149-152.

Bhargava, V. K. *Medicinal uses and pharmacological properties of Crocus sativus linn (saffron). International Journal of Pharmacy and Pharmaceutical Science*, 2011. *3*(Suppl 3), 2226.

Dhar, A., Mehta, S., Dhar, G., Dhar, K., Banerjee, S., Van Veldhuizen, P., . . . Banerjee, S. K. *Crocetin inhibits pancreatic cancer growth. Molecular Cancer Therapeutics*, 2009. *8*(3), 711.

Golmohammadi, F. *Saffron and its farming, economic importance, export, medicinal characteristics and various uses in South Khorasan Province – East of Iran. International Journal Farming and Allied Sciences*, 2014. *3*(5), 566-596.

Hosseinzadeh, H., & Ghenaati, J. *Evaluation of the antitussive effect of stigma and petals of saffron (Crocus sativus) and its components, safranal and crocin in guinea pigs. Fitoterapi*, 2006. *77*(6), 446-448.

Hosseinzadeh, H., & Jahanian, Z. Effect of *Crocus sativusL. (saffron) stigma and its constituents, crocin and safranal, on morphine withdrawal syndrome in mice. Phytotherapy Research*, 2010. *24*(5), 726-730.

Hosseinzadeh, H., & Nassiri-Asl, M. *Avicenna's (Ibn Sina) the canon of medicine and saffron (Crocus sativus): A review. Phytotherapy Research*, 2013. *27*(4), 475-483.

Hosseinzadeh, H., & Noraei, N. B. *Anxiolytic and hypnotic effect of Crocus sativus aqueous extract and its constituents, crocin and safranal, in mice. Phytotherapy Research*, 2009. *23*(6), 768-774.

Hosseinzadeh, H., Ziaee, T., & Sadeghi, A. *The effect of saffron, Crocus sativus stigma, extract and its constituents, safranal and crocin on sexual behaviors in normal male rats. Phytomedicine,* 2008. *15*(6-7), 491-495.

Imenshahidi, M., Hosseinzadeh, H., & Javadpour, Y. *Hypotensive effect of aqueous saffron extract (Crocus sativus L.) and its constituents, safranal and crocin, in normotensive and hypertensive rats. Phytotherapy Research,* 2010. *24*(7), 990-994. doi: 10.1002/ptr.3044.

Karimi, E., Oskoueian, E., Hendra, R., & Jaafar, H. Z. *Evaluation of Crocus sativus L. stigma phenolic and flavonoid compounds and its antioxidant activity. Molecules, 2010. 15(9), 6244-6256.*

Ordoudi, S. A., Befani, C. D., Nenadis, N., Koliakos, G. G., & Tsimidou, M. Z. *Further examination of antiradical properties of Crocus sativus stigmas extract rich in crocins. Journal of Agriculture and Food Chemistry,* 2009. *57*(8), 3080-3086.

Papandreou, M. A., Kanakis, C. D., Polissiou, M. G., Efthimiopoulos, S., Cordopatis, P., Margarity, M., & Lamari, F. N. *Inhibitory activity on amyloid-beta aggregation and antioxidant properties of Crocus sativus stigmas extract and its crocin constituents. Journal of Agriculture and Food Chemistry,* 2006. *54*(23), 8762-8768.

Poma, A., Fontecchio, G., Carlucci, G., & Chichiriccò, G. *Anti-inflammatory properties of drugs from saffron crocus. Anti-Inflammatory Anti-Allergy Agents Medicinal Chemistry,* 2012. *11*(1), 37-51.

Raja, A. S. M., Pareek, P. K., Shakyawar, D. B., Wani, S. A., Nehvi, F. A., & Sofi, A. H. *Extraction of natural dye from saffron flower waste and its application on pashmina fabric. Advances in Applied Science Research,* 2012. *3*(1), 156-161.

Serrano-Díaz, J., Sánchez, A. M., Maggi, L., Martínez-Tomé, M., García-Diz, L., Murcia, M. A., & Alonso, G. L. *Increasing the applications of Crocus sativus flowers as natural antioxidants. Journal of Food Science,* 2012. *77*(11), C1162-C1168.

Srivastava, R., Ahmed, H., Dixit, R. K., Dharamveer, & Saraf,

S. A. *Crocus sativus* L.: *A comprehensive review. Pharmacognosy Review*, 2010. *4*(8), 200-208.

ONYCHA

Barros, L. et al. *Antifungal activity and detailed chemical characterization of Cistus ladanifer phenolic extracts. Industrial Crops and Products*, 2013. *41*, 41-45.

Bousta, D. et al. *Phytochemical screening, antidepressant and immunomodulatory effects of aqueous extract of Cistus ladanifer l. From Morocco. International Journal of Phytopharmacology*, 2013. *4*(1), 12-17.

Yadav, Y., & Singh, R. *Screening of mineral elements in Cistus ladanifer and Cistus libanotis essential oils and their leaves. Oriental Journal of Chemistry*, 2013. *29*(4).

COSTUS

Ambawade, S. D., Mhetre, N. A., Muthal, A. P., & Bodhankar, S. L. *Pharmacological evaluation of anticonvulsant activity of root extract of Saussurea lappa in mice. European Journal of Integrative Medicine*, 2009. *1*(3), 131-137.

Choi, Y. K., Cho, S-G., Woo, S-W., Woo, S-M., Yun, Y-J., Jo, J., . . . Ko, S-G. *Saussurea lappa Clarke-derived costunolide prevents TNFa-induced breast cancer cell migration and invasion by inhibiting NF-κB activity. Evidence-Based Complementary and Alternative Medicine*, 2013. 936257.

Hasson, S. S. A., Al-Balushi, M. S., Alharthy, K., Al-Busaidi, J. Z., Aldaihani, S., Othman, M. S., . . . Ahmedldris, M. *Evaluation of anti-resistant activity of Auklandia (Saussurea lappa) root against some human pathogens. Asian Pacific Journal of Tropical Biomedicine*, 2013. *3*(7), 557-562.

Kim, H. R., Kim, J. M., Kim, M. S., Hwang, J. K., Park, Y. J., Yang, S. H., . . . Lee, Y. R. *Saussurea lappaextract suppresses TPA-induced cell invasion via inhibition of NF-κB-dependent MMP-9 expression in MCF-7 breast cancer cells. BMC Complementary and Alternative Medicine*, 2014. *14*, 170.

Ko, S. G., Kim, H. P., Jin, D. H., Bae, H. S., Kim, S. H., Park, C. H., & Lee, J. W. Saussurea lappa induces G2-growth arrest and apoptosis in AGS gastric cancer cells. *Cancer Letters*, 2005. *220*, 11-19.

Madhuri, K. Elango, K., & Ponnusankar, S. *Saussurea lappa(Kuth root): Review of its traditional uses, phytochemistry and pharmacology. Oriental Pharmacy and Experimental Medicine*, 2011. *12*(1), 1-9.

Pandey, M. M., Rastogi, S., & Rawat, A. K. *Saussurea costus: Botanical, chemical and pharmacological review of an ayurvedic medicinal plant. Journal of Ethnopharmacology*, 2007. *110*(3), 379-390.

Saleem, T. S., Lokanath, N., Prasanthi, A., Madhavi, M., Mallika, G., & Vishnu, M. N. *Aqueous extract of Saussurea lappa root ameliorate oxidative myocardial injury induced by isoproterenol in rats. Journal of Advanced Pharmaceutical Technology and Research*, 2013. *4*(2), 94-100.

Shoji, N., Umeyama, A., Saito, N., Takemoto, T., Kajiwara, A., & Ohizumi, Y. *Vasoactive Substances from Saussurea lappa. Journal of Natural Products*, 1986. *49*(6), 1112–1113.

Sutar, N., Garai, R., Sharma, U. S., Singh, N., & Roy, S. D. *Antiulcerogenic activity of Saussurea lappa root. International Journal of Pharmacy and Life Sciences*, 2011. *2*(1), 516-520.

Thara, K. M., & Zuhra, K. F. *Comprehensive in-vitro pharmacological activities of different extracts of Saussurea lappa. European Journal of Experimental Biology*, 2012. *2*(2), 417-420.

Waly, N. M. *Verifying the scientific name of Costus [Saussurea lappa ((Decne.) C.B. Clarke.) – Asteraceae). JKAU: Science*, 2009. *21*(2), 327-334.

HENNA

Abulyazid, I. Mahdy, E. M. E., & Ahmed, R. M. *Biochemical study for the effect of henna (Lawsonia inermis) on Escherichia coli. Arabian Journal of Chemistry*, 2013. *6*(3), 265-273.

Alam, M. M., Rahman, M. L., & Haque, M. Z. *Extraction of henna leaf dye and its dyeing effects on textile fibre. Bangladesh Journal of Scientific and Industrial Research*, 2007. *42*(2), 217-222.

Babili, F. E., Valentin, A., & Chatelain, C. *Lawsonia inermis: Its anatomy and its antimalarial, antioxidant and human breast cancer cells MCF7 activities. Pharmaceutica Analytica Acta,* 2013.4(1). doi: 10.4172/2153-2435.1000203

Chandra Kalyan Reddy, Y., Sandya, L., Sandeep, D., Ruth Salome, K., Nagarjuna, S., & Padmanabha Reddy, Y. *Evaluation of diuretic activity of aqueous and ethanolic extracts of Lawsonia inermis* leaves in rats. *Asian Journal of Plant Science Research*, 2011. *1*(3), 28-33.

Chaudhary, G., Goyal, S., & Poonia, P. *Lawsonia inermisLinnaeus:A phytopharmacological review. International Journal of Pharmaceutical Sciences and Drug Research*, 2010. *2*(2), 91-98.

Dasgupta, T., Rao, A. R., & Yadava, P. K. *Modulatory effect of henna leaf (Lawsonia inermis) on drug metabolising phase I and phase II enzymes, antioxidant enzymes, lipid peroxidation and chemically induced skin and forestomach papillomagenesis in mice. Molecular and Cellular Biochemistry*, 2003. *245*, 11-22.

Hossein, C. M., Maji, H. S., & Chakraborty, P. *Hepatoprotective activity of Lawsonia inermis Linn, warm aqueous extract in carbon tetrachloride induced hepatic injury in Wister rats. Asian Journal of Pharmaceutical and Clinical Research*, 2011. *4*(3), 106-109.

Kapadia, G. J. Rao, G. S., Sridhar, R., Ichiishi, E., Takasaki, M., Suzuki, N., . . . Tokuda, H. *Chemoprevention of skin cancer: Effect of Lawsonia inermis L. (Henna) leaf powder and its pigment artifact, lawsone in the Epstein-Barr virus early antigen activation assay and in two-*

stage mouse skin carcinogenesis models. Anticancer Agents in Medicinal Chemistry, 2013. *13*(10), 1500-1507.

Kidanemariam, T. K., Tesema, T. K., Asressu, K. H., & Boru, A. D. *Chemical investigation of Lawsonia inermis L. leaves from Afar Region, Ethiopia. Oriental Journal of Chemistry*, 2013. *29*(3).

Nayak, B. S., Isitor, G., Davis, E. M., & Pillai, G. K. *The evidence based wound healing activity of Lawsonia inermis Linn. Phytotherapy Research*, 2007. *21*(9), 827-831.

Owis, A. S. *An economical dyeing process for cotton, polyester and cotton/polyester blended fabrics. Journal of Textile Management*, 2010. *6*(4).

Scientific Committee on Consumer Safety (SCCS). Opinion on Lawsonia inermis (Henna), 2013. COLIPA C169. SCCS/1511/13. Retrieved from: http://ec.europa.eu/health/scientific_committees/consumer_safety/docs/sccs_o_140.pdf

CHAPTER IV – SACRED TREES

Dafni, A. *On the present-day veneration of sacred trees in the holy land. Folklore*, 2011. *48*, 7-30.

CEDARWOOD

Devmurari, V. P. *Antibacterial evaluation of ethanolic extract of Cedrus deodara wood. Applied Science Research*, 2010. *2*(2), 179-183.

Hudson, J., Kuo, M., & Vimalanathan, S. *The antimicrobial properties of cedar leaf (Thuja plicata) oil; a safe and efficient decontamination agent for buildings. International Journal of Environmental Research and Public Health*, 2011. *8*(12), 4477-4487.

Kumar, M., Qadri, M., Sharma, P. R., Kumar, A., Andotra, S. S., Kaur, T., & Shah, B. A. *Tubulin inhibitors from an endophytic fungus isolated from Cedrus deodara. Journal of Natural Products*, 2013. *76*(2), 194-199.

Patil, S., Prakash, T., Kotresha, D., Rama Rao, N., & Pandy, N. *Antihyperlipidemic potential of Cedrus deodara extracts in monosodium glutamate induced obesity in neonatal rats. Indian Journal of Pharmacology,* 2011. *43*(6), 644-647.

Shinde, U. A., Phadke, A. S., Mungantiwar, A. A., Dikshit, V. J., & Saraf, M. N. *Preliminary studies on the immunomodulatory activity of Cedrus deodara oil. Fitoterapia,* 1999. *70*(4), 333-339.

Shinde, U. A., Phadke, A. S., Nair, A. M., Mungantiwar, A. A., Dikshit, V. J., & Saraf, M. N. *Studies on the anti-inflammatory and analgesic activity of Cedrus deodara. Journal of Ethnopharmcology,* 1999. *65*, 21-27.

Singh, S. K., Shanmugavel, M., Kampasi, H., Singh, R., Mondhe, D. M., Rao, J. M., . . . Qazi, G. N. *Cedrus deodara stem having anticancer activity. Planta Medica,* 2007. *73*(6), 519-526.

Tiwari, A. K., Srinivas, P. V., Kumar, S. P., & Rao, J. M. *Heart of Cedrus deodara shows free radical scavenging (antioxidant) activity. Journal of Agricultural and Food Chemistry,* 2001. *49*, 4642.

DATE PALM

Aamir, J., Kumari, A., Khan, M. N., & Medam, S. K. *Evaluation of the combinational antimicrobial effect of Annona squamosa and Phoenix dactylifera seeds methanolic extract on standard microbial strains. International Research Journal of Biological Sciences,* 2013. *2*(5), 68-73.

Abdelrahman, H. A. *Protective effect of dates (Phoenix dactylifera L.) and licorice (Glycyrrhiza glabra) on carbon tetrachloride-induced hepatotoxicity in dogs. Global Veterinaria,* 2012. *9*(2), 184-191.

Al-Qarawi, A. A., Mousa, H. M., Ali, B. E. H., Abdel-Rahman, H., & El-Mougy, S. A. *Protective effect of extracts from dates (Phoenix dactylifera L.) on carbon tetrachloride-induced hepatotoxicity in rats. International Journal of Applied Research in Veterinary Medicine,* 2004. *2*(3), 176-180.

Al-Taher, A. Y. *Anticonvulsant effects of 3, 4-dimethoxy toluene, the major constituent of Phoenix dactylifera L Spathe in mice. Scientific Journal of King Faisal University (Basic and Applied Sciences),* 2008. *9*(2), 1429.

Bircher, W. H. *The date palm: A boon for mankind.* Cairo, Egypt: Cairo University Herbarium, 1990.

Bokhari, N. A., & Perveen, K. *In vitro inhibition potential of Phoenix dactylifera L. extracts on the growth of pathogenic fungi. Journal of Medicinal Plant Research,* 2012. *6*(6), 1083-1088.

Darby, J. W., Ghalioungi, P., & Louis, G. *Food: The gift of Osiris,* 2 vols. London, New York: Academic Press, 1977.

Ismail, W. I. W., & Radzi, M. N. F. M. *Evaluation on the benefits of date palm (Phoenix dactylifera) to the brain. Alternative and Integrative Medicine,* 2013. *2*(4). doi: 10.4172/2327-5162.1000115.

Morton, J. *Fruits of warm climates.* Miami, FL: Echo Point Books and Media, 1987.

Njagi, J. M., Piero, M. N., Ngeranwa, J. J. N., Njagi, E. N. M., Kibiti, C. M., Njue, W. M., . . . Gathumbi, P. K. *Assessment of antidiabetic potential of Ficus sycomorus on alloxan-induced diabetic mice. International Journal of Diabetes Research,* 2012. *1*(4), 47-51.

Okwuosa, C. N., Udeani, T. K., Umeifekwem, J. E., Onuba, A. C., Anioke, I. C., & Madubueze, R. E. *Hepatoprotective effect of methanolic fruit extracts of Phoenix dactylifera (arecaceae) on thioacetamide induced liver damage in rats. American Journal of Phytomedicine and Clinical Therapeutics,* 2014. *2*(3), 290-300.

Pujari, R. R., Vyawahare, N. S., & Kagathara, V. G. *Evaluation of antioxidant and neuroprotective of date palm Phoenix dactylifera against bilateral common carotid artery occulusion in rats. Indian Journal of Experimental Biology,* 2011. *49*(8), 627-633.

Rahmani, A., Aly, S. M., Ali, H., Babiker, A. Y., Srikar, S., & Khan, A. A. *Therapeutic effects of date fruits (Phoenix dactylifera) in the prevention of diseases via modulation of anti-inflammatory, anti-oxidant and anti-tumour activity. International Journal of Clinical and Experimental Medicine,* 2014. *7*(3), 483-491.

Sandabe, U. K., Onyeyili, P. A., & Chibuzo, G. A. *Sedative and anticonvulsant effects of aqueous extract of Ficus sycomorus L. (Moraceae) stembark in rats. Veterinarski Arhiv*, 2003. *73*(2), 103-110.

Vayalil, P. K. *Antioxidant and antimutagenic properties of aqueous extract of date fruit (Phoenix dactylifera L. arecaceae). Journal of Agricultural and Food Chemistry*, 2002. *50*(3), 610-617.

Vayalil, P. K. Date fruits (*Phoenix dactyliferaLinn): An emerging medicinal food. Critical Reviews in Food Science and Nutrition,* 2012. 52(3), 249-271.

Vembu, S., Sivanasan, D., & Prasanna, G. *Effect of Phoenix dactylifera on high fat diet induced obesity. Journal of Chemical and Pharmaceutical Research*, 2012. *4*(1), 348-352.

OLIVE

Abut, E., Guveli, H., Yasar, B., Bolukbas, C., Bolukbas, F. F. Ince, A. T., . . . Kurdas, O. O. *Administration of olive oil followed by a low volume of polyethylene glycol-electrolyte lavage solution improves patient satisfaction with right-side colonic cleansing over administration of the conventional volume of polyethylene glycol-electrolyte lavage solution for colonoscopy preparation. Gastrointestinal Endoscopy*, 2009. *70*(3), 515-521.

Badía-Tahull, M. B., Llop-Talaverón, J. M., Leiva-Badosa, E., Biondo, S., Farran-Teixidó, L. Ramón-Torrell, J. M., & Jódar-Masanes, R. *A randomised study on the clinical progress of high-risk elective major gastrointestinal surgery patients treated with olive oil-based parenteral nutrition with or without a fish oil supplement. British Journal of Nutrition*, 2010. *104*(5), 737-741.

Berbert, A. A., Kondo, C. R., Almendra, C. L., Matsuo, T., & Dichi, I. *Supplementation of fish oil and olive oil in patients with rheumatoid arthritis. Nutrition*, 2005. *21*(2), 131-136.

Bermudez, B., Lopez, S., Ortega, A., Varela, L. M., Pacheco, Y. M., Abia, R., & Muriana, F. J. *Oleic acid in olive oil: From a metabolic framework toward a clinical perspective. Current Pharmaceutical Design*, 2011. *17*(8), 831-843.

Bogani, P., Galli, C., Villa, M., & Visioli, F. *Postprandial anti-inflammatory and antioxidant effects of extra virgin olive oil. Atherosclerosis*, 2007. *190*(1), 181-186.

Chiu, C. C., Su, K. P., Cheng, T. C., Liu, H. C., Chang, C. J., Dewey, M. E., . . . Huang, S. Y. *The effects of omega-3 fatty acids monotherapy in Alzheimer's disease and mild cognitive impairment: A preliminary randomized double-blind placebo-controlled study. Progress in Neuro-psychopharmacology and Biological Psychiatry*, 2008. *32*(6), 1538-1544.

Cicero, A. F., Nascetti, S., López-Sabater, M. C., Elosua, R., Salonen, J. T., Nyyssönen, K., . . . *EUROLIVE Study Group. Changes in LDL fatty acid composition as a response to olive oil treatment are inversely related to lipid oxidative damage: The EUROLIVE study. Journal of American College of Nutrition*, 2008. *27*(2), 314-320.

de la Lastra Romero, C. A. *An up-date of olive oil and bioactive constituents in health: Molecular mechanisms and clinical implications. Current Pharmaceutical Design*, 2011. *17*(8), 752-753.

Delgado-Lista, J., Garcia-Rios, A., Perez-Martinez, P., Lopez-Miranda, J., & Perez-Jimenez, F. *Olive oil and haemostasis: Platelet function, thrombogenesis and fibrinolysis. Current Pharmaceutical Design*, 2011. *17*(8), 778-785.

Ferrara, L. A., Raimondi, S., d'Episcopo, L., Guida, L., Dello Russo, A., & Marotta, T. *Olive oil and reduced need for antihypertensive medications. Archives of Internal Medicine*, 2000. *160*, 837-842.

Fitó, M., Cladellas, M., de la Torre, R., Martí, J., Alacántara, M., Pujadas-Bastardes, M., . . . *members of the SOLOS investigators. Antioxidant effect of virgin olive oil in patients with stable coronary heart disease: A randomized, crossover, controlled, clinical trial. Atherosclerosis*, 2005. *181*(1), 149-158.

Fitó, M., Cladellas, M., de la Torre, R., Martí, J., Muñoz, D., Schröder, H., . . . SOLOS Investigators. *Anti-inflammatory effect of virgin olive oil in stable coronary disease patients: A randomized, crossover,* controlled trial. *European Journal of Clinical Nutrition*, 2008. *62*(4), 570-574.

Fleming, H. P., Walter, W. M. Jr, & Etchells, J. L. *Antimicrobial properties of oleuropein and products of its hydrolysis from green olives. Applied Microbiology*, 1973. *26*(5), 777-782.

Göbel, Y., Koletzko, B., Böhles, H. J., Engelsberger, I., Forget, D., Le Brun, A., . . . Zimmerman, A. *Parenteral fat emulsions based on olive and soybean oils: a randomized clinical trial in preterm infants. Journal of Pediatric Gastroenterological Nutrition*, 2003. *37*(2), 161-167.

Huschak, G., Zur Nieden, K., Hoell, T., Riemann, D., Mast, H., & Stuttmann, R. *Olive oil based nutrition in multiple trauma patients: A pilot study. Intensive Care Medicine*, 2005. *31*(9), 1202-1208.

Kiechl-Kohlendorfer, U., Berger, C., & Inzinger, R. *The effect of daily treatment with an olive oil/lanolin emollient on skin integrity in preterm infants: A randomized controlled trial. Pediatric Dermatology*, 2008. *25*(2), 174-178.

Lucas, L., Russell, A., & Keast, R. *Molecular mechanisms of inflammation. Anti-inflammatory benefits of virgin olive oil and the phenolic compound oleocanthal. Current Pharmaceutical Design*, 2011. *17*(8), 754-768.

Machowetz, A., Gruendel, S., Garcia, A. L., Harsch, I., Covas, M. I., Zunft, H. J., & Koebnick, C. *Effect of olive oil consumption on serum resistin concentrations in healthy men. Hormone and Metabolism Research*, 2008. *40*(10), 697-701.

Marrugat, J., Covas, M. I., Fitó, M., Schröder, H., Miró-Casas, E., Gimeno, E., . . . SOLOS Investigators. *Effects of differing phenolic content in dietary olive oils on lipids and LDL oxidation – A randomized controlled trial. European Journal of Nutrition*, 2004. *43*(3), 140-147.

Olsen, S. F., Østerdal, M. L., Salvig, J. D., Mortensen, L. M., Rytter, D., Secher, N. L., & Henriksen, T. B. *Fish oil intake compared with olive oil intake in late pregnancy and asthma in the offspring:*

16 y of registry-based follow-up from a randomized controlled trial. American Journal of Clinical Nutrition, 2008. *88*(1), 167-175.

Onar, P., Yildiz, B. D., Yildiz, E. A., Besler, T., & Abbasoglu, O. *Olive oil-based fat emulsion versus soy oil-based fat emulsion in abdominal oncologic surgery. Nutrition in Clinical Practice*, 2011. *26*(1), 61-65.

Pérez-Martínez, P., García-Ríos, A., Delgado-Lista, J., Pérez-Jiménez, F., & López-Miranda, J. *Mediterranean diet rich in olive oil and obesity, metabolic syndrome and diabetes mellitus. Current Pharmaceutical Design*, 2011.*17*(8), 769-777.

Perona, J. S., Cañizares, J., Montero, E., Sánchez-Domínguez, J. M., & Ruiz-Gutiérrez, V. *Virgin olive oil reduces blood pressure in hypertensive elderly subjects. Clinical Nutrition*, 2004. *23*(5), 1113-1121.

Pretty, I. A., Gallagher, M. J., Martin, M. V., Edgar, W. M., & Higham, S. M. *A study to assess the effects of a new detergent-free, olive oil formulation dentifrice in vitro and in vivo. Journal of Dentistry*, 2003. *31*(5), 327-332.

Razquin, C., Martinez, J. A., Martinez-Gonzalez, M. A., Mitjavila, M. T., Estruch, R., & Marti, A. A. *A 3 years follow-up of a Mediterranean diet rich in virgin olive oil is associated with high plasma antioxidant capacity and reduced body weight gain. European Journal of Clinical Nutrition*, 2009. *63*(12), 1387-1393.

Ruano, J., López-Miranda, J., de la Torre, R., Delgado-Lista, J., Fernández, J., Caballero, J., & Jiménez, F. *Intake of phenol-rich virgin olive oil improves the postprandial prothrombotic profile in hypercholesterolemic patients. American Journal of Clinical Nutrition*, 2007. *86*(2), 341-346.

Samieri, C., Féart, C., Proust-Lima, C., Peuchant, E., Tzourio, Stapf, D., . . . Barberger-Gateau, P. *Olive oil consumption, plasma oleic acid, and stroke incidence: The Three-City Study. Neurology*, 2011. *77*(5), 418-425.

St-Onge, M. P., Lamarche, B., Mauger, J. F., & Jones, P. J. *Consumption of a functional oil rich in phytosterols and medium-chain triglyceride oil improves plasma lipid profiles in men. Journal of Nutrition,* 2003. *133*(6), 1815-1820.

Sutherland, W. H. F., de Jong, S. A., Walker, R. J., Williams, M. J. A., Skeaff, C. M., Duncan, A., & Harper, M. *Effect of meals rich in heated olive and safflower oils on oxidation of postprandial serum in healthy men. Atherosclerosis,* 2002. *160*(1), 195-203.

Tranter, H. S., Tassou, S. C., & Nychas, G. J. *The effect of the olive phenolic compound, oleuropein, on growth and enterotoxinB production byStaphylococcus aureus. Journal of Applied Bacteriology,* 1993. *74*(3), 253-259.

Verallo-Rowell, V. M., Dillague, K. M., & Syah-Tjundawan, B. S. *Novel antibacterial and emollient effects of coconut and virgin olive oils in adult atopic dermatitis. Dermatitis,* 2008. *19*(6), 308-315.

Visioli, F., Caruso, D., Grande, S., Bosisio, R., Villa, M., Galli, G., . . . Galli, C. *Virgin Olive Oil Study (VOLOS): Vasoprotective potential of extra virgin olive oil in mildly dyslipidemic patients. European Journal of Nutrition,* 2005. *44*(2), 121-127.

Visioli, F., Poli, A., & Gall, C. *Antioxidant and other biological activities of phenols from olives and olive oil. Medical Research Review,* 2002. *22*(1), 65-75.

Webb, A. N., Hardy, P., Peterkin, M., Lee, O., Shalley, H., Croft, K. A., . . . Bines, J. E. *Tolerability and safety of olive oil-based lipid emulsion in critically ill neonates: A blinded randomized trial. Nutrition,* 2008. *24*(11-12), 1057-1064.

Zwingle, E. *Olive oil: Elixir of gods. National Geographic,* 1999. *196*(3).

POMEGRANATE

Abram, M. *The pomegranate: Sacred, secular, and sensuous symbol of ancient Israel. Studia Antiqua,* 2009. *7*(1), 23-33.

Adeel, S., Ali, S., Bhatti, I. A., & Zsila, F. *Dyeing of cotton fabric* using pomegranate (Punica granatum) aqueous extract. Asian Journal of Chemistry, 2009. 21, 3493-3499.

Adhami, V. Q., Khan, N., & Mukhtar, H. Cancer chemoprevention by pomegranate: Laboratory and clinical evidence. Nutrition and Cancer, 2009. 6, 811-815.

Afaq, F., Zaid, M. A., Khan, N., Dreher, M., & Mukhtar, H. Protective effect of pomegranate-derived products on UVB-mediated damage in human reconstituted skin. Experimental Dermatology, 2009. 18, 553-561.

Ahangari, B., & Sargolzaei, J. Extraction of pomegranate seed oil using subcritical propane and supercritical carbon dioxide. Theoretical Foundations of Chemical Engineering, 2012.46(3), 258-265.

Al-Zoreky, N. S. Antimicrobial activity of pomegranate (Punica granatum L.) fruit peels. International Journal of Food Microbiology, 2009. 134, 244-248.

Amin, A. R. M. R., Kucuk, O., Khuri, F. R., & Shin, D. M. Perspectives for cancer prevention with natural compounds. Journal of Clinical Oncology, 2009. 27, 2712-2725.

Aviram, M., & Dornfeld, L. Pomegranate juice consumption inhibits serum angiotensin converting enzyme activity and reduces systolic blood pressure. Atherosclerosis, 2001. 158(1), 195-198.

Babu, U. V., Mitra, S. K., Saxena, E., & Suriyanarayanan, R. Composition, used to prevent dental diseases e.g. plaque, comprises extracts ofPunica granatum, Acacia arabica, Terminalia chebula, Terminalia bellerica, Emblica oficinalis and Embelia ribes, and naturally derived excipients e.g. xylitol. Patent numbers: US2009185987-A1; IN200800167-I1, 2009.

Bagri, P., Ali, M., Aeri, V., Bhowmik, M., & Sultana, S. Antidiabetic effect of Punica granatum flowers: Effect on hyperlipidemia, pancreatic cells lipid peroxidation and antioxidant enzymes in experimental diabetes. Food Chemistry and Toxicology, 2009. 47, 50-54.

Bhowmik, D., Gopinath, H., Kumar, B. P., Duraivel, S., Aravind, G., & Kumar, K. P. S. *Medicinal uses of Punica granatum and its health benefits. Pharmacognosy*, 2013. *1*(5), 28-35.

Bialonska, D., Kasimsetty, S. G., Khan, S. I., & Ferreira, D. *Urolithins, intestinal microbial metabolites of Pomegranate ellagitannins, exhibit potent antioxidant activity in a cell-based assay. Journal of Agricultural and Food Chemistry*, 2009. *57*, 10181-10186.

Bialonska, D., Kasimsetty, S. G., Schrader, K. K., & Ferreira, D. *The effect of pomegranate (Punica granatum L.) by-products and ellagitannins on the growth of human gut bacteria. Journal of Agricultural and Food Chemistry*, 2009. *57*, 8344-8349.

Briese, M., Ghosh, R., Oezka, Y., & Weiss, T. Cosmetic use of an active agent mixture, obtained from e.g. *Clintonia borealis* or *Punica granatum*, for preventing and/or inhibiting the effect (that is, nonpathological effect) of psychoemotional stress on the hair. Patent number: DE102009043486-A1, 2010.

Caligiani, A., Bonzanini, F., Palla, G., Cirlini, M., & Bruni, R. *Characterization of a potential nutraceutical ingredient: pomegranate (Punica granatum L.) seed oil unsaponifiable fraction. Plant Foods for Human Nutrition*, 2010. *65*(3), 277-283.

Celik, I., Temur, A., & Isik, I. *Hepatoprotective role and antioxidant capacity of pomegranate (Punica granatum) flowers infusion against trichloroacetic acid-exposed in rat. Food Chemistry and Toxicology*, 2009. *47*, 145-149.

Cho, G., Kim, D., Kim, E., Kim, H., Kim, S., Moon, E., . . . Park, C. *Skin external composition useful for preventing skin dryness and skin aging, comprises extracts of Punica granatum and Tussilago farfara*. Patent number: KR2010031839-A, 2010.

Cuccioloni, M., Mozzicafreddo, M., Sparapani, L., Spina, M., Eleuteri, A. M., Fioretti, E., & Angeletti, M. *Pomegranate fruit components modulate human thrombin. Fitoterapia*, 2009. *80*, 301-305.

Dell'Agli, M., Galli, G. V., Corbett, Y., Taramelli, D., Lucantoni, L., Habluetzel, A., . . . Bosisio, E. *Antiplasmodial activity of Punica granatum L. fruit rind. Journal of Ethnopharmacology*, 2009. *125*, 279-285.

Desai, A. *Herbal formulation for treating sickle cell disease.* Patent number: IN200801962-I3, 2010.

Endo, E. H., Cortéz, D. A., Ueda-Nakamura, T., Nakamura, C. V., & Dias Filho, B. P. *Potent antifungal activity of extracts and pure compound isolated from pomegranate peels and synergism with fluconazole againstCandida albicans. Research in Microbiology*, 2010. *161*(7), 534-540.

Grossmann, M. E., Mizuno, N. K., Schuster, T., & Cleary, M. P. *Punicic acid is an ω-5 fatty acid capable of inhibiting breast cancer proliferation. International Journal of Oncology*, 2010. *36*, 421-426.

Guo, G., Wang, H. X., & Ng, T. B. *Pomegranin, an antifungal peptide from pomegranate peels. Protein Peptide Letters*, 2009. *16*, 82-85.

Hadipour-Jahromy, M., & Mozaffari-Kermani, R. *Chondroprotective effects of pomegranate juice on monoiodoacetate-induced osteoarthritis of the knee joint of mice. Phytotherapy Research*, 2010. *24*, 182-185.

Haidari, M., Ali, M., Ward Casscells, S., 3rd, & Madjid, M. *Pomegranate (Punica granatum) purified polyphenol extract inhibits influenza virus and has a synergistic effect with oseltamivir. Phytomedicine*, 2009. *16*(12), 1127-1136.

Hartman, R. E, Shah, A., Fagan, A. M., Schwetye, K. E., Parsadanian, M., Schulman, R. N., . . . Holtzman, D. M. *Pomegranate juice decreases amyloid load and improves behaviour in a mouse model of Alzheimer's Disease. Neurobiology of Disease*, 2006. *24*(3), 506-515.

Jadeja, R. N., Thounaojam, M. C., Patel, D. K., Devkar, R. V., & Ramachandran, A. V. *Pomegranate (Punica granatum L.) juice supplementation attenuates isoproterenol-induced cardiac necrosis in rats. Cardiovascular Toxicology*, 2010. *10*, 174-180.

Kasimetty, S. G., Bialonska, D., Reddy, M. K., Thornton, C., Willett, K. L., & Ferreira, D. *Effects of pomegranate chemical constituents/intestinal microbial metabolites on CYP1B1 in 22Rv1 prostate cancer cells. Journal of Agricultural and Food Chemistry*, 2009. *57*, 10636-10644.

Khan, N., Afaq, F., Kweon, M. H., Kim, K., & Muktar, H. *Oral Consumption of Pomegranate Fruit Extract Inhibits Growth and Progression of Primary Lung Tumors in Mice. Cancer Research*, 2007. *67*(7), 3475-3482.

Khan, S. A. *The role of pomegranate (Punica granatum L.) in colon cancer. Pakistan Journal of Pharmaceutical Sciences*, 2009. *22*, 346-348.

Kulkarni, S. S., Gokhale, A. V., Bodake, U. M., & Pathade, G. R. *Cotton dyeing with natural dye extracted from pomegranate (Punica granatum) peel. Universal Journal of Environmental Research and Technology*, 2011. *1*(2), 135.

Lansky, E. P., & Newman, R. A. *Punica granatum (pomegranate) and its potential for prevention and treatment of inflammation and cancer. Journal of Ethnopharmacology*, 2007. *109*, 177-206.

Lee, C. J., Chen, L. G., Liang, W. L., & Wang, C. C. *Anti-inflammatory effects of Punica granatum Linne in vitro and in vivo. Food Chemistry*, 2010. *118*, 315-322.

Li, Y., Qi, Y., Huang, T. H. W., Yamahara, J., & Roufogalis, B. D. *Pomegranate flower: A unique traditional antidiabetic medicine with dual PPAR-a/-γ activator properties. Diabetes, Obesity and Metabolism*, 2008. *10*, 10-17.

Menezes, S. M., Cordeiro, L. N., & Viana, G. S. *Punica granatum (pomegranate) extract is active against dental plaque. Journal of Herbal Pharmacotherapy*, 2006. *6*(2), 79-92.

Miguel, M. G., Neves, M. A., & Antunes, M. D. *Pomegranate (Punica granatum L.): A medicinal plant with myriad biological properties – A short review. Journal of Medicinal Plants Research*, 2010. *4*(25), 2836-2847.

Neurath, A. R., Strick, N., Li, Y. Y., & Debnath, A. K. *Punica granatum(pomegranate) juice provides an HIV-1 entry inhibitor and candidate topical microbicide. BMC Infectious Disease*, 2004. *4*, 41.

Pantuck, A. J., Leppert, J. T., Zomorodian, N., Aronson, W., Hong, J., Barnard, R. J., . . . Belidegrun, A. *Phase II study of pomegranate juice for men with rising prostate-specific antigen following surgery or radiation for prostate cancer. Clinical Cancer Research*, 2006. *12*(13), 4018-4026.

Settar, S., & Korisettar, R. (Eds.) *Indian archaeology in retrospect. II. Protohistory. The archaelogy of Indus Valley civilization.* Indian Council of Historical Research. New Delhi: Manohar, 2002.

Singh, K., Jaggi, A. S., & Singh, N. *Exploring the ameliorative potential of Punica granatum in dextran sulphate sodium induced ulcerative colitis in mice. Phytotherapy Research*, 2009. *23*, 1565-1574.

Sturgeon, S. R., & Ronnenberg, A. G. *Pomegranate and breast cancer: Possible mechanisms of prevention. Nutrition Reviews*, 2010. *68*(2), 122-128.

Su, X., Sangster, M. Y., & D'Souza, D. H. *In vitro effects of pomegranate juice and pomegranate polyphenols on foodborne viral surrogates. Foodborne Pathogens and Disease*, 2010. *7*(12), 1473-1479.

WILLOW

Aronson, S. M. *The miraculous willow tree. Rhode Island Medical Journal,* 1994. *77*(6), 159-161.

Beaver, W. (1980). *Analgesic development: A brief history and perspective. Journal of Clinical Pharmacology, 20*(4), 213-215.

Bottero, J. *Everyday life in ancient Mesopotamia.* Baltimore, MD:John Hopkins University Press, 2001.

Breasted, J. H. *The Edwin Smith surgical papyrus.* Chicago: University of Chicago Press, 1930.

Brock, W. *The biochemical tradition. In W. F. Bynum & R. Porter*

(Eds.), *Companion encyclopaedia of the history of medicine.* London: Routledge, 1993.

Butler, R. N. *Thanks Hippocrates, for the first miracle drug. Geriatrics,* 1998. *53*(1), 15.

Highfield, E. S., & Kemper, K, J. *White willow bark. Longwood Herbal Task Force,* 1999.

Jeffreys, D. *Aspirin: The remarkable story of a wonder drug.* New York, London: Bloomsbury, 2004.

Klein, R. *The 'fever bark' tree. Natural History,* 1976. *85*, 10-19.

Lloyd, G. E. R. (Ed.) *Hippocratic writings.* Hardmondsworth, UK: Penguin, 1978.

Maclagan, T. J. *The treatment of rheumatism by salicin and salicylic acid. British Medical Journal,* 1876. *1*(803), 627.

Mahdi, J. G., *Medicinal potential of willow: A chemical perspective of aspirin discovery. Journal of Saudi Chemical Society,* 2010. *14*(3), 317-322.

Nunn, J. E. *Ancient Egyptian medicine.* London: British Museum Press, 1996.

Porter, R. *The greatest benefit to mankind: A medical history of humanity from antiquity to the present.* London: Harper Collins, 1997.

Stone, E. An account of the success of the bark of the willow in the cure of agues. *Philosophical Transactions,* 1763. *(1683-1775), 53*(1763), 195-200.

MYRTLE

Alipour, G. Dashti, S., & Hosseinzadeh, H. *Review of pharmacological effects of Myrtus communis L. and its active constituents. Phytotherapy Research,* 2014. 28(8), 1125-1136.

Dogan, A. *Investigations Myrtus communis L. plant's volatile oil yield, their physical-chemical properties and their compositions.* Ankara, Turkey: Ankara University, Agricultural Faculty Press, 1978.

Gençler Özkan, A. M., & Gençler Güray, Ç. A *Mediterranean: Myrtus communis l. (myrtle). In J-P. Morel, & Mercuri, A. M. Plants and culture: Seeds of the cultural heritage of Europe.* Centro Eurpeo per I Beni Culturali Ravello, Edipuglia Bari, 2009.

Hayder, N., Abdelwahed, A., Kilani, S., Ben Ammar, R., Mahmoud, A., Ghedira, K., & Chekir-Ghedira, L. *Anti-genotoxic and free-radical scavenging activities of extracts from (Tunisian) Myrtus communis. Mutation Research/Genetic Toxicology and Environmental Mutagenesis,* 2004. 564(1), 89-95.

Mehrabani, M., Kazemi, A., Mousavi, S. A. A., Rezaifar, M., Alikhah, H., & Nosky, A. *Evaluation of antifungal activities of Myrtus communis L. by bioautography method. Jundishapur Journal of Microbiology,* 2013. 6(8), e8316.

Ozek, T., Demirci, B., & Baser, K. H. *Chemical composition of Turkish myrtle oil. Journal of Essential Oil Research,* 2000. 12,541-544.

Qaraaty, M., Kamali, S. H., Dabaghain, F. H., Zafarghanghi, N., Mokaberinejad, R., Mobli, M., . . . Talei, D. *Effect of myrtle fruit syrup on abnormal uterine bleeding: A randomized double-blind, placebo-controlled pilot study. DARU Journal of Pharmaceutical Sciences,* 2014. 22(45). doi:10.1186/2008-2231-22-45.

Rahimmalek, M., Mirzakhani, M., & Pirbalouti, A. G. *Essential oil variation among 21 wild myrtle (Myrtus communis L.) populations collected from different geographical regions in Iran. Industrial Crops and Products,* 2013. 51, 328-333.

Serce, S., Ercisli, S., Sengul, M., Gunduz, K., & Orhan, E. *Antioxidant activities and fatty acid composition of wild grown myrtle (Myrtus communis L.) fruits. Pharmacognosy Magazine,* 2010. 6(21), 9-12.

Sumbul, S., Ahmad, M. A., Asif, M., & Akhtar, M. *Myrtus communis Linn. – A review. Indian Journal of Natural Products and Resources,* (2011). 2(4), 395-402.

CHAPTER V – HEALING AND CULINARY HERBS

Aboelsoud, N. H. Herbal medicine in ancient Egypt. *Journal of Medicinal Plants Research*, 2010. *4(2)*, 82-86.

AbouZid, S. F., & Mohamed, A. A. *Survey on medicinal plants and spices used in Beni-Sueif, Upper Egypt. Journal of Ethnobiology and Ethnomedicine*, 2011. *7*(18). doi: 10.1186/1746-4269-7-18.

Azaizeh, H., Saad, B., Khalil, K., & Said, O. *The state of the art of traditional Arab herbal medicine in the eastern region of the Mediterranean: A review. Evidence Based Complementary and Alternative Medicine*, 2006. *3*(2), 229-235.

Jouanna, J. *Greek medicine from Hippocrates to Galen: Selected papers.* Leiden, The Netherlands: Koninklijke Brill, 2012 .

Mininberg, D. T. *The legacy of ancient Egyptian medicine. In J. P. Allen (Ed.), The art of medicine in ancient Egypt* (13-15). New York: Metropolitan Museum Press, 2005.

Newmyer, S. T. *Asaph's 'book of remedies': Greek science and Jewish apologetics. Sudhoffs Archiv*, 1992. *76*(1), 28-36.

Nunn, J. F. *Ancient Egyptian medicine.* Norman, OK: University of Oklahoma Press, 1996.

Saad, B., Azaizeh, H., & Said, O. *Tradition and perspectives of Arab herbal medicine: A review. Evidence Based Complementary and Alternative Medicine*, 2005. *2*(4), 475-479.

HYSSOP

Al-Bandak, G., & Oreopoulou, V. *Antioxidant properties and composition of Majorana syriaca extracts. European Journal of Lipid Science Technology*, 2007. *109*, 247-255.

Džamić, A. M., Soković, M. D., Novaković, M., Jadranin, M., Ristić, M. S., Tešević, V., & Marin, P. D. *Composition, antifungal and antioxidant properties of Hyssopus officinalis L. subsp. pilifer (Pant.) Murb. essential oil and deodorized extracts. Industrial Crops and Products*, 2013. *51*, 401-407.

Fathiazad, F., & Sanaz, H.*A review on Hyssopus officinalis L.: Composition and biological activities. African Journal of Pharmacy and Pharmacology*, 2011. *5*(17), 1959-1966.

Fleisher, A., & Fleisher, Z. *Identification of biblical hyssop and origin of the traditional use of oregano-group herbs in the Mediterranean region. Economic Botany*, 1988. *42*(2), 232-241.

Ghfir, B., Fonvielle, J. L., & Dargent, R. *Influence of essential oil of Hyssopus officinalis on the chemical composition of the walls of Aspergillus fumigatus* (Fresenius). *Mycopathologia*, 1997. *138*(1), 7-12.

Hirobe, C., Qiao, Z-S., Takeya., & Itokawa, H. *Cytotoxic principles from Majorana syriaca. Natural Medicines,* 1998.*52*(1), 74-77.

Kamal, H. *Encyclopedia of Islamic medicine.* Cairo: General Egyptian Book Organization, 1975.

Kizil, S., Haşimi, N., Tolan, V., Kilininç, E., & Karataş, H. *Chemical composition, antimicrobial and antioxidant activities of hyssop (Hyssopus officinalis L.) essential oil. Notulae Botanicae Horti Agrobotanici Cluj-Napoca*, 2010. *38*(3), 99-103.

Levey, M. (Trans.). *Aqrabadhin of Al-Kindi.* Madison, WI: University of Wisconsin Press, 1966.

Levey, M. *Early Arabic pharmacology.* Leiden, Netherlands: E. J. Brill, 1973.

Lu, M., Battinelli, L., Daniele, C., Melchioni, C., Salvatore, G., & Mazzanti, G. *Muscle relaxing activity of Hyssopus officinalis essential oil on isolated intestinal preparations. Planta Medica*, 2002. *68*(3), 213-216.

Mitić, V., & Đorđević, S. *Essential oil composition of Hyssopus officinalis L. cultivated in Serbia. Facta Universitatis Series: Physics, Chemistry and Technology*, 2000. *2*(2), 105-108.

Miyazaki, H., Matsuura, H., Yanagiya, C., Mizutani, J., Tsuji, M., & Ishihara, C. *Inhibitory effects of hyssop (Hyssopus officinalis) extracts on intestinal alpha-glucosidase activity and postprandial hyperglycemia. Journal of Nutrition Science and Vitaminology (Tokyo)*, 2003. *49*(5), 346-349.

Saleh Abu-Lafi, S., Odeh, I., Dewik, D., Qabajah, M., Hanus, L. O., & Dembitsky, V. M. *Thymol and carvacrol production from leaves of wild Palestinian Majorana syriaca. Bioresource Technology*, 2008. *99*(9), 3914-3918.

Savage-Smith, E. *Islamic culture and the medical arts.* Bethesda, MD: National Library of Medicine, 1994.

Siddiqi, M. Z. *Studies in Arabic and Persian medical literature.* Calcutta: Calcutta University Press, 1959.

Usama, I. S. (Narr.). (n.d.) *Sunna Abu-Dawud, book 28, no. 3846 (Part of the Hadith, a narrative record of the sayings of Mohammed and his companions).*

WORMWOOD

Fiamegos, Y. C., Kastritis, P. L., Exarchou, V., Han, H., Bonvin, A. M. J. J., Vervoort, J., . . . Tegos, G. P. *Antimicrobial and efflux pump inhibitory activity of caffeoylquinic acids from Artemisia absinthium* against Gram-positive pathogenic bacteria. *PLoS ONE*, 2011. *6*(4), e18127.

Lachenmeier, D. W. Wormwood (*Artemisia absinthium* L.) – *A curious plant with both neurotoxic and neuroprotective properties? Journal of Ethnopharmacology*, 2010. *131*(1), 224-227.

Singh, R., Verma, P. K., & Singh, G. *Total phenolic, flavonoids and tannin contents in different extracts of Artemisia absinthium. Journal of Intercultural Ethnopharmacology*, 2012. *1*(2), 101-104.

Zafab, M. M., Hamdard, M. E., & Hameed, A. *Screening of Artemisia absinthium for antimalarial effects on Plasmodium berghei* in mice: A preliminary report. *Journal of Ethnopharmacology*, 1990. *30*(2), 223-226.

RUE

Diwan, R., Shinde, A., & Malpathak, N. *Phytochemical composition and antioxidant potential of Ruta graveolens* L. in vitro culture lines. *Journal of Botany*, 2012. 685427.

Freyer, G., You, B., Villet, S., Tartas, S., Fournei-Federico, C., Trillet-Lenoir, V., . . . Falandry, C. *Open-label uncontrolled pilot study to evaluate complementary therapy with Ruta graveolens 9c in patients with advanced cancer. Homeopathy*, 2014. *103*(4), 232-238.

Halvaei, I., Roodsari, H. R., & Harat, Z. N. *Acute effects of Ruta graveolens L. on sperm parameters and DNA integrity in rats. Journal of Reproductive Infertility*, 2012. *13*(1), 33-38.

Nauman, I. T., Hamad, M. N., & Hussain, S. A. *Comparative study of the analgesic activity of two Iraqi medicinal plants, Ruta graveolens and Matricaria chamomilla extracts. Journal of Intercultural Ethnopharmacology*, 2012. *1*(2), 79-83.

Madari, H., & Jacobs, R. S. *An analysis of cytotoxic botanical formulations used in the traditional medicine of ancient Persia as abortifacients. Journal of Natural Products*, 2004. *67*(8), 1204-1210.

Pandey, P., Mehta, A., & Hajra, S. *Evaluation of antimicrobial activity of Ruta graveolens stem extracts by disc diffusion method. Journal of Phytology*, 2011. *3*(3), 92-95.

Pollio, A., De Natale, A., Appetit, E., Aliotta, G., & Touwaide, A. *Continuity and change in the Mediterranean medical tradition: Ruta spp. (rutaceae) in Hippocratic medicine and present practices. Journal of Ethnopharmacology*, 2008. *116*(3), 469-482.

Preethi, K. C., Kuttan, G., & Kuttan, R. *Anti-tumour activity of Ruta graveolens extract. Asian Pacific Journal of Cancer Prevention*, 2006. *7*(3), 439-443.

Raghav, S. K., Gupta, B., Agrawai, C., Goswami, K., & Das, H. R. *Anti-inflammatory effect of Ruta graveolens L. in murine macrophage cells. Journal of Ethnopharmacology*, 2006. *104*(1-2), 234-239.

CORIANDER

Al-Suhaimi, E. A. (n.d.). *Effect of Coriandrum sativum, a common herbal medicine, on endocrine and reproductive organ structure and function. The Internet Journal of Alternative Medicine*, *7*(2).

Burdock, G. A., & Carabin, I. G. *Safety assessment of coriander (Coriandrum sativum L.) essential oil as a food ingredient. Food and Chemical Toxicology*, 2009. *47*(1), 22-34.

Chandan, H. S., Tapas, A. R., & Sakarkar, D. M. *Anthelmintic activity of extracts of Coriandrum sativum linn. In Indian earthworm. International Journal of Phytomedicine*, 2011. *3*, 36-40.

Diederichsen, A *Coriander (*Coriandrum sativum *L.). Promoting the conservation and use of underutilized and neglected crops. 3.* Gatersleben, Germany; Rome: Institute of Plant Genetics and Crop Plant Research; International Plant Genetic Resources Institute, 1996.

Deepa, B., & Anuradha, C. V. *Antioxidant potential of Coriandrum sativum L. seed extract. Indian Journal of Experimental Biology*, 2011. *49*(1), 30-38.

Dhanapakiam, P., Joseph, J. M., Ramaswamy, V. K., Moorthi, M., & Kumar, A. S. *The cholesterol lowering property of coriander seeds (Coriandrum sativum): Mechanism of action. Journal of Environmental Biology*, 2008. *29*(1), 53-56.

Koppula, S., & Choi, D. K. *Anti-stress and anti-amnesic effects of Coriandrum sativum Linn (umbelliferae) extract – An experimental study in rats. Tropical Journal of Pharmaceutical Research*, 2012. *11*(1), 36-42.

McGovern, P. E., Mirzoian, A., & Hall, G. R. *Ancient Egyptian herbal wines. Proceedings of National Academy of Sciences of the United States of America*, 2009. *106*(18), 7361-7366.

Minija, J., & Thoppil, J. E. *Volatile oil constitution and microbicidal activities of essential oils of Coriandrum sativumL. Journal of Natural Remedies*, 2001. *1*(2), 147-150.

Nair, V., Singh, S., & Gupta, Y. K. *Evaluation of disease modifying activity of Coriandrum sativum in experimental models. Indian Journal of Medical Research*, 2012. *135*, 240-245.

Naquvi, K. J., Ali, M., & Ahmad, J. *Two new aliphatic lactones from the fruits of Coriandrum sativum L. Organic and Medicinal Chemistry Letters*, 2012. *16*(2), 28.

Rajeshwari, C. U., Siri, S., & Andallu, B. *Antioxidant and antiarthritic potential of coriander (Coriandrum sativum L.) leaves.e-SPEN Journal,* 2012. *7*(6), e223-e228.

Ramadan, M. M., Algader, N. N. E. A., El-kamali, H. H., Ghanem, K. Z., & Farrag, A. R. H. *Chemopreventive effect of Coriandrum sativum fruits on hepatic toxicity in male rats. World Journal of Medical Science,* 2013. *8*(4), 322-333.

Sahib, N. G., Anwar, F., Gilani, A. H., Hamid, A. A., Saari, N., & Alkharfy, K. M. *Coriander (Coriandrum sativum L.): A potential source of high-value components for functional foods and nutraceuticals – A review. Phytotherapy Research,* 2013. *27*(10), 1439-1456.

Waheed, A., Miana, G. A., Ahmad, S. I., & Khan, M. A. *Clinical investigation of hypoglycemic effect of Coriandrum sativum in type-2 (NIDDM) diabetic patients. Pakistan Journal of Pharmacology,* 2006. *23*(1), 7-11.

CUMIN

Andallu, B., & Ramya, V. *Antihyperglycemic, cholesterol-lowering and HDL-raising effects of cumin (Cuminum cyminum) ceeds in type-2 diabetes. Journal of Natural Remedies,* 2007. *7*(1).

Bettaieb, I., Bourgou, S., Wannes, W. A., Hamrouni, I., Limam, F., & Marzouk, B. *Essential oils, phenolics, and antioxidant activities of different parts of cumin (Cuminum cyminum L.). Journal of Agricultural and Food Chemistry,* 2010. *58*(19), 10410-10418.

Bokaeian, M., Shiri, Y., Bazi, S., Saeidi, S., & Sahi, Z. *Antibacterial activities of Cuminum cyminum Linn essential oil against multi-drug resistant Escherichia coli. International Journal of Infection,* 2014. *1*(1), e18739.

Derakhshan, S., Sattari, M., & Bigdeli, M. *Effect of cumin (Cuminum cyminum) seed essential oil on biofilm formation and plasmid Integrity of Klebsiella pneumoniae. Pharmacognosy Magazine,* 2010. *6*(21), 57-61.

El-Said, A. H. M. & Goder, E-H. *Antifungal activities of Cuminum cyminum and Pimpinella anisum essential oils. International Journal of Current Microbiology and Applied Sciences*, 2014. *3*(3), 937-944.

Gohari, A. R., & Saeidnia, S. *A review on phytochemistry of Cuminum cyminum seeds and its standards from field to market. Pharmacognosy Journal*, 2011. *3*(25), 1-5.

Kalaivani, P., Saranya, R. B., Ramakrishnan, G., Ranju, V., Sathiya, S., Gayathri, V., . . . Thanikachalam, S. *Cuminum cyminum, a dietary spice, attenuates hypertension via endothelial nitric oxide synthase and NO pathway in renovascular hypertensive rats. Clinical and Experimental Hypertension*, 2013. *35*(7), 534-542.

Kumar, A. *Protective affect of Cuminum cyminum and Coriandrum sativum on profenofos induced liver toxicity. International Journal of Pharmaceutical and Biological Archives*, 2011. *2*(5), 1405-1409.

Milan, K. S. M., Dholakia, H., Tiku, P. K., & Vishveshwaraiah, P. *Enhancement of digestive enzymatic activity by cumin (Cuminum cyminum L.) and role of spent cumin as a bionutrient. Food Chemistry*, 2008. *110*(3), 678-683.

Nadeem, M., & Riaz, A. Cumin (*Cuminum cyminum*) *as a potential source of antioxidants. Pakistan Journal of Food Science*, 2012. *22*(2), 101-107.

Poole, F. 'Cumin, set milk, honey': *An ancient Egyptian medicine container (Naples 828). The Journal of Egyptian Archaeology*, 2001. *87*, 175-180.

Prakash, E., & Gupta, D. K. Cytotoxic activity of ethanolic extract of *Cuminum cyminum* Linn against seven human cancer cell line. *Universal Journal of Agricultural Research*, 2014. *2*(1), 27-30.

Sahoo, H. B., Sahoo, S. K., Sarangi, S. P., Sagar, R., & Kori, M. L. *Anti-diarrhoeal investigation from aqueous extract of Cuminum cyminum Linn. seed in albino rats. Pharmacognosy Research*, 2014. *6*(3), 204-209.

Salari, S., Khosravi, A. R., Katiraee, F., Ayatollahi Mousavi, S. A. Shokri, H., & Nikbakht Borujeni, G. H. *Evaluation of inhibitory* effects of *cuminum cyminum* oil on the fluconazaole resistant and susceptible Candida albicans isolated from HIV patients in Iran. Journal of American Science, 2012. *8*(5).

Sayyah, M., Mahboubi, A., & Kamalinejad, M. *Anticonvulsant effect of the fruit essential oil of Cuminum cyminum in mice. Pharmaceutical Biology,* 2002. *40*(6), 478-480.

Willatgamuwa, S. A., Platel, K., Saraswathi, G., & Srinivasan, K. *Antidiabetic influence of dietary cumin seeds (Cuminum cyminum) in streptozotocin induced diabetic rats. Nutrition Research,* 1998. *18*(1), 131-142.

FITCHES OR BLACK CUMIN

Ahmad, H., Khan, I., & Nisar, W. *Antioxidation and antiglycation properties of Bunium bulbocastanum fruits various fractions and its possible role in reducing diabetes complication and ageing. Vitamins and Minerals,* 2014. *3*(1). doi: 10.4172/vms.1000118.

Ait Mbarek, L., Ait Mouse, H., Elabbadi, N., Bensalah, M., Gamouh, A., Aboufatima, R., . . . Zyad, A. *Anti-tumor properties of blackseed (Nigella sativa L.) extracts. Brazilian Journal of Medicinal and Biological Research,* 2007. *40*(6), 839-847.

Akhondian, J., Kianifar, H., Raoofziaee, M., Moayedpour, A., Toosi, M. B., & Khajedaluee, M. *The effect of thymoquinone on intractable pediatric seizures (pilot study). Epilepsy Research,* 2011. *93*(1), 39-43.

Al-Jenoobi, F. I., Al-Thukair, A. A., Abbas, F. A., Ansari, M. J., Alharfy, K. M., Al-Mohizea, A. M., . . . Jamil, S. *Effect of black seed on dextromethorphan O- and N-demethylation in human liver microsomes and healthy human subjects. Drug Metabolism Letters,* 2010. *4*(1), 51-55.

Badary, O. A., Al-Shabanah, O. A., Nagi, M. N., Al-Rikabi, A. C., & Elmazar, M. M. *Inhibition of benzo(a)pyrene-induced forestomach carcinogenesis in mice by thymoquinone. European Journal of Cancer Prevention,* 1999. *8*(5), 435-440.

Bamosa, A. O., Kaatabi, H., Lebdaa, F. M., Elq, A. M., & Al-Sultana, A. *Effect of Nigella sativa seeds on the glycemic control of patients with type 2 diabetes mellitus. Indian Journal of Physiology and Pharmacology*, 2010. *54*(4), 344-354.

Boskabady, M. H., Javan, H., Sajady, M., & Rakhshandeh, H. *The possible prophylactic effect of Nigella sativa seed extract in asthmatic patients. Fundamentals of Clinical Pharmacology*, 2007. *21*(5), 559-566.

Cemek, M., Enginar, H., Karaca, T., & Unak, P. *In vivo radioprotective effects of Nigella sativa L oil and reduced glutathione against irradiation-induced oxidative injury and number of peripheral blood lymphocytes in rats. Photochemistry and Photobiology*, 2006. *82*(6), 1691-1696.

Chakravarty, N. *Inhibition of histamine release from mast cells by nigellone. Annals of Allergy, Asthma, and Immunology*, 1993. *70*(3), 237-242.

Dada, M. H., & Abdel-Rahman, M. S. *Hepatoprotective activity of thymoquinone in isolated rat hepatocytes. Toxicology Letters*, 1998. *95*(1), 23-29.

Dehkordi, F. R., & Kamkhah, A. F. *Antihypertensive effect of Nigella sativa seed extract in patients with mild hypertension. Fundamentals of Clinical Pharmacology*, 2008. *22*(4), 447-452.

Effenberger-Neidnicht, K., & Schobert, R. *Combinatorial effects of thymoquinone on the anti-cancer activity of doxorubicin. Cancer Chemotherapy and Pharmacology*, 2011. *67*(4), 867-874.

El-Abhar, H. S., Abdallah, D. M., & Saleh, S. *Gastroprotective activity of Nigella sativa oil and its constituent, thymoquinone, against gastric mucosal injury induced by ischaemia/reperfusion in rats. Journal of Ethnopharmacology*, 2003. *84*(2-3), 251-258.

El Tahir, K. E., Ashour, M. M., & al-Harbi, M. M. *The cardiovascular actions of the volatile oil of the black seed (Nigella sativa) in rats: Elucidation of the mechanism of action. General Pharmacology*, 1993. *24*(5), 1123-1131.

Gali-Muhtasib, H., Diab-Assaf, M., Boltze, C., Al-Hmaira, J., Hartig, R., Roessner, A., & Schneider-Stock, R. *Thymoquinone extracted from black seed triggers apoptotic cell death in human colorectal cancer cells via a p53-dependent mechanism. International Journal of Oncology*, 2004. *25*(4), 857-866.

Gheita, T. A., & Kenawy, S. A. *Effectiveness of Nigella sativa oil in the management of rheumatoid arthritis patients: A placebo controlled study. Phytotherapy Research*, 2012. *26*(8), 1246-1248.

Ghosheh, O. A., Houdi, A. A., & Crooks, P. A. *High performance liquid chromatographic analysis of the pharmacologically active quinones and related compounds in the oil of the black seed (Nigella sativa L.). Journal of Pharmaceutical and Biomedical Analysis*, 1999. *19*(5), 757-762.

Haq, A., Lobo, P. I., Al-Tufail, M., Rama, N. R., & Al-Sedairy, S. T. *Immunomodulatory effect of Nigella sativa proteins fractionated by ion exchange chromatography. International Journal of Immunopharmacology*, 1999. *21*(4), 283-295.

Houghton, P. J., Zarka, R., de las Heras, B., & Hoult, J. R. *Fixed oil of Nigella sativa and derived thymoquinone inhibit eicosanoid generation in leukocytes and membrane lipid peroxidation. Planta Medica*, 1995. *61*(1), 33-36.

Iddamaldeniya, S. S., Thabrew, M. I., Wickramasinghe, S. M., Ratnatunge, N., & Thammitiyagodage, M. G. *A long-term investigation of the anti-hepatocarcinogenic potential of an indigenous medicine comprised of Nigella sativa, Hemidesmus indicus and Smilax glabra. Journal of Carcinogenesis*, 2006. *5*(11).

Islam, S. N., Begum, P., Ahsan, T., Huque, S., & Ahsan, M. *Immunosuppressive and cytotoxic properties of Nigella sativa. Phytotherapy Research*, 2004. *18*(5), 395-398.

Kalus, U., Pruss, A., Bystron, J., Jurecka, M., Smekalova, A., Lichius, J. J., & Kiesewetter, H. *Effect of Nigella sativa (black seed) on subjective feeling in patients with allergic diseases. Phytotherapy Research*, 2003. *17*(10), 1209-1214.

Khader, M., Bresgen, N., & Eckl, P. M. *In vitro toxicological properties of thymoquinone. Food and Chemical Toxicology*, 2009. *47*(1), 129-133.

Khan, I., Ahmad, H., Ali, N., Ahmad, B., & Tanoli, H. *Screening of Bunium bulbocastanum for antibacterial, antifungal, phytotoxic and haemagglutination activities. Pakistan Journal of Pharmceutical Sciences,*(2013. *26*(4), 787-791.

Mohamed, A. M., Metwally, N. M., & Mahmoud, S. S. *Sativa seeds against Schistosoma mansoni different stages. Memórias do Instituto Oswaldo Cruz,* 2005. *100*(2), 205-211.

Salem, E. M., Yar, T., Bamosa, A. O., Al-Quorain, A., Yasawy, M. I., Alsulaiman, R. M., & Ranshawa, M. A. *Comparative study of Nigella sativa and triple therapy in eradication of Helicobacter pylori in patients with non-ulcer dyspepsia. Saudi Journal of Gastroenterology,* 2010. *16*(3), 207-214.

Steinmann, A., Schatzle, M., Agathos, M., & Breit, R. *Allergic contact dermatitis from black cumin (Nigella sativa) oil after topical use. Contact Dermatitis,* 1997. *36*(5), 268-269.

Zaoui, A., Cherrah, Y., Alaoui, K., Mahassine, N., Amarouch, H., & Hassar, M. (2002). Effects of *Nigella sativa* fixed oil on blood homeostasis in rat. *Journal of Ethnopharmacology, 79*(1), 23-26.

Zaoui, A., Cherrah, Y., Mahassini, N., Alaoui, K., Amarouch, H., & Hassar, M. *Acute and chronic toxicity of Nigella sativa fixed oil. Phytomedicine,* 2002. *9*(1), 69-74.

DILL

Al-Snafi, A. E. *The pharmacological importance of Anethum graveolens. A review. International Journal of Pharmacy and Pharmaceutical Science,* 2014. *6*(4), 11-13.

Bahramikia, S., & Yazdanparast, R. *Antioxidant and free radical scavenging activities of different fractions of Anethum graveolens leaves using in vitro models. Pharmacologyonline,* 2008. *2*, 219-233.

Kaur, G. J., & Arora, D. S *Antibacterial and phytochemical screening of Anethum graveolens, Foeniculum vulgare and Trachyspermum ammi. BMC Complementary and Alternative* Medicine, 2009. *9*(30). doi:10.1186/1472-6882-9-30.

Sahib, A. S., Mohammad, I. H., & Al-Gareeb, A. I. Effects of *Anethum graveolens* leave powder on lipid profile in hyperlipidemic patients. *Spatula DD*, 2012. *2*(3), 153-158.

Sharopov, F. S., Wink, M., Gulmurodov, I. S., Isupov, S. J., Zhang, H., & Setzer, W. N. *Composition and bioactivity of the essential oil of Anethum graveolens from Tajikistan. International Journal of Medicinal and Aromatic Plants*, 2013. *3*(2), 125-130.

Singh, G., Maurya, S., de Lampasona, M. P., & Catalan, C. *Chemical constituents, antimicrobial investigations, and antioxidative potentials of* Anethum graveolens L. *essential oil and acetone extract: Part 52. Journal of Food Science*, 2005. *70*, M208–M215.

Stavri, M., & Gibbons, S. *The antimycobacterial constituents of dill* (Anethum graveolens*). Phytotherapy Research*, 2005. *19*, 938-941.

Tian, J., Ban, X., Zeng, H., He, J., Chen, Y., & Wang, Y. *The mechanism of antifungal action of essential oil from dill (Anethum graveolens L.) on Aspergillus flavus. PLoS ONE, 2012. 7(1), e30147.* doi: 10.1371 / journal.pone.0030147.

Zagami, S. E., Golmakani, N., Kabirian, M., & Shakeri, M. T. *Effect of dill seed (Anethum graveolens) in uterus contraction pattern in active phase of labor. Indian Journal of Traditional Knowledge*, 2012. *11*(4), 602-606.

MUSTARD

Kiasalari, Z., Khalili, M., Roghani, M., & Sadeghian, A. *Antiepileptic and antioxidant effect of Brassica nigra on pentylenetetrazol-induced kindling in mice. Iran Journal of Pharmaceutical Research*, 2012. *11*(4), 1209-1217.

Nozhat, F., Alaee, S., Behzadi, K., & Chegini, N. A. *Evaluation of possible toxic effects of spearmint (Mentha spicata) on the reproductive system, fertility and number of offspring in adult male rats. Avicenna Journal of Phytomedicine*, 2014. *4*(6), 420-429.

Saharkhiz, M. J., Motamedi, M., Zomorodian, K., Pakshir, K., Miri, R., & Hemyari, K. *Chemical composition, antifungal and antibiofilm activities of the essential oil of Mentha piperita L.ISRN Pharmaceutics*, 2012. 718645.

Stoin, D., Radu, F., Poiana, M-A., & Dugaru, D. *Antibacterial activity of isothiocyanates, active principles in Brassica nigra seeds (IV).* Universitatea de Ştiinţe Agricole şi Medicină Veterinară Iaşi, 2007.

Taher, Y. A. *Antinociceptive activity of Mentha piperita leaf aqueous extract in mice. Libyan Journal of Medicine*, 2012. *7*, 16205. doi: 10.3402/ljm.v7i0.16205.

Tayarani-Najaran, Z., Talasaz-Firoozi, E., Nasiri, R., Jalali, N., & Hassanzadeh, M. K. *Antiemetic activity of volatile oil from Mentha spicata and Mentha × piperita in chemotherapy-induced nausea and vomiting. Ecancer*, 2013. *7*(290). doi: 10.3332/ecancer.2013.290.

Thirumalai, T., Therasa, S. V., Elumalai, E. K., & David, E. *Hypoglycemic effect of Brassica juncea (seeds) on streptozotocin induced diabetic male albino rat. Asian Pacific Journal of Tropical Biomedicine*, 2011). *1*(4), 323-325.

MINT

Alalli, H., Chikhi, H., Dib, M. E. A., Muselli, A., Fekih, N., Meliani, N., . . . Costa, J. *Antioxidant activity and chemical analysis of Mentha spicata cultivated from west northern region of Algeria by headspace solid phase micro-extraction and hydro-distillation. Natural Products*, 2013. *9*(6), 258-263.

Alankar, S. *A review on peppermint oil. Asian Journal of Pharmaceutical and Clinical Research*, 2009. *2*(2), 27-33.

Alyaa, S. J. *Antibacterial activity of oils extracts of Brassica nigra seeds on some bacteria isolated from plaque and healthy teeth in children (1-5) years. Basrah Journal of Science (B)*, 2012. *30*(1), 105-119.

Barbalho, S. M., Machado, F. M. V. F., Oshiiwa, M., Abreu, M., Guiger, E. L., Tomazela, P., & Goulart, R. A. *Investigation of the effects of peppermint (Mentha piperita) on the biochemical and anthropometric profile of university students. Ciência e Tecnologia de Alimentos*, 2011. *31*(3), 584-588.

Bhupesh, G., Amutha, C., Nandagopal, S., Ganeshkumar, A., Sureshkumar, P., & Saravana Murali, K. *Antibacterial activity of Mentha piperita L. (peppermint) from leaf extracts – a medicinal plant. Acta agriculturae Slovenica*, 2007. *89*(1), 73-79.

Chakraborty, P. S., Singh, J. P., Rai, M. K., Singh, P., Vichitra, A. K., Singh, A. K. N., . . . Siddiqui, V. A. *Mentha piperita– A multicentric clinical verification study conducted by CCRH. Indian Journal of Research in Homoeopathy*, 2008. *2*(4), 26-33.

I could not find this in the text., E., Chabir, R., Taouil, R., & Senhaji, O. *In-vitro antioxidant activity and GC/MS studies on the leaves of Mentha piperita (Lamiaceae) from Morocco. International Journal of Pharmaceutical Sciences and Drug Research*, 2011. *3*(2), 130-136.

Gupta, S. *Hepatoprotective effects from the leaf extracts of Brassica juncea in CCl4 induced rat model. Der Pharmacia Sinica*, 2011. *2*(4), 274-285.

Hajighasemi, F. *Cytotoxic effect of Mentha spicata aqueous extract on cancerous cell lines in vitro. Journal of Medicinal Plants Research*, 2011. *5*(20), 5142-5147.

Herro, E., & Jacob, S. E. *Mentha piperita(peppermint). Dermatitis*, 2010. *21*(6), 327-329.

Isücan, G., Kirimer, N., Kürkcüoğlu, M., Başer, K. H., & Demirci, F. *Antimicrobial screening of Mentha piperita essential oils. Journal of Agricultural and Food Chemistry*, 2002. *50*(14), 3943-3946.

Jeyakumar, E., Lawrence, R., & Pal, T. *Comparative evaluation in the efficacy of peppermint (Mentha piperita) oil with standards antibiotics against selected bacterial pathogens. Asian Pacific Journal of Tropical Biomedicine,* 2011. S253-S257.

Karousou, R., Balta, M., Hanlidou, E., & Kokkini, S. *"Mints", smells and traditional uses in Thessaloniki (Greece) and other Mediterranean countries. Journal of Ethnopharmacology,* 2007. *109*(2), 248-257.

Kaushik, P., Mathur, M., Rawat, N., Saxena, T., Mobar, S., & Meena, P. D. *Study of Mentha piperita against gamma radiation in mice. Oxidants and Antioxidants in Medical Science,* 2013. *2*(4), 285-295.

Kazemi, M., Rostami, H., & Shafiei, S. *Antibacterial and antifungal activity of some medicinal plants from Iran. Journal of Plant Sciences,* 2012. *7*, 55-66.

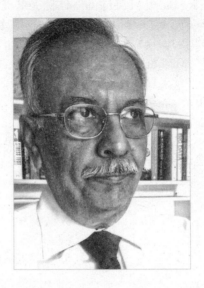

Sudhir Ahluwalia started his career in the Indian Forest Service office. After twenty three years in forestry, he spent the next ten years in the technology industry, first as a business consultant with Tata Consultancy Services, and then as adviser to multiple tech companies. Currently, he is a columnist, writing articles related to technology and natural products. *Holy Herbs* is his second book. Connect with Sudhir at www.sudhirahluwalia.com